OCE-13   OCCUPATIONAL COMPETENCY EXAM SERIES

This is your
PASSBOOK for...

Cosmetology

Test Preparation Study Guide
Questions & Answers

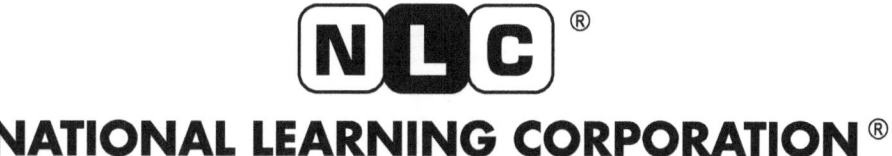

COPYRIGHT NOTICE

This book is SOLELY intended for, is sold ONLY to, and its use is RESTRICTED to individual, bona fide applicants or candidates who qualify by virtue of having seriously filed applications for appropriate license, certificate, professional and/or promotional advancement, higher school matriculation, scholarship, or other legitimate requirements of education and/or governmental authorities.

This book is NOT intended for use, class instruction, tutoring, training, duplication, copying, reprinting, excerption, or adaptation, etc., by:

1) Other publishers
2) Proprietors and/or Instructors of "Coaching" and/or Preparatory Courses
3) Personnel and/or Training Divisions of commercial, industrial, and governmental organizations
4) Schools, colleges, or universities and/or their departments and staffs, including teachers and other personnel
5) Testing Agencies or Bureaus
6) Study groups which seek by the purchase of a single volume to copy and/or duplicate and/or adapt this material for use by the group as a whole without having purchased individual volumes for each of the members of the group
7) Et al.

Such persons would be in violation of appropriate Federal and State statutes.

PROVISION OF LICENSING AGREEMENTS – Recognized educational, commercial, industrial, and governmental institutions and organizations, and others legitimately engaged in educational pursuits, including training, testing, and measurement activities, may address request for a licensing agreement to the copyright owners, who will determine whether, and under what conditions, including fees and charges, the materials in this book may be used them. In other words, a licensing facility exists for the legitimate use of the material in this book on other than an individual basis. However, it is asseverated and affirmed here that the material in this book CANNOT be used without the receipt of the express permission of such a licensing agreement from the Publishers. Inquiries re licensing should be addressed to the company, attention rights and permissions department.

All rights reserved, including the right of reproduction in whole or in part, in any form or by any means, electronic or mechanical, including photocopying, recording, or by any information storage and retrieval system, without permission in writing from the Publisher.

Copyright © 2025 by
National Learning Corporation

212 Michael Drive, Syosset, NY 11791
(516) 921-8888 • www.passbooks.com
E-mail: info@passbooks.com

PASSBOOK® SERIES

THE *PASSBOOK® SERIES* has been created to prepare applicants and candidates for the ultimate academic battlefield – the examination room.

At some time in our lives, each and every one of us may be required to take an examination – for validation, matriculation, admission, qualification, registration, certification, or licensure.

Based on the assumption that every applicant or candidate has met the basic formal educational standards, has taken the required number of courses, and read the necessary texts, the *PASSBOOK® SERIES* furnishes the one special preparation which may assure passing with confidence, instead of failing with insecurity. Examination questions – together with answers – are furnished as the basic vehicle for study so that the mysteries of the examination and its compounding difficulties may be eliminated or diminished by a sure method.

This book is meant to help you pass your examination provided that you qualify and are serious in your objective.

The entire field is reviewed through the huge store of content information which is succinctly presented through a provocative and challenging approach – the question-and-answer method.

A climate of success is established by furnishing the correct answers at the end of each test.

You soon learn to recognize types of questions, forms of questions, and patterns of questioning. You may even begin to anticipate expected outcomes.

You perceive that many questions are repeated or adapted so that you can gain acute insights, which may enable you to score many sure points.

You learn how to confront new questions, or types of questions, and to attack them confidently and work out the correct answers.

You note objectives and emphases, and recognize pitfalls and dangers, so that you may make positive educational adjustments.

Moreover, you are kept fully informed in relation to new concepts, methods, practices, and directions in the field.

You discover that you are actually taking the examination all the time: you are preparing for the examination by "taking" an examination, not by reading extraneous and/or supererogatory textbooks.

In short, this PASSBOOK®, used directedly, should be an important factor in helping you to pass your test.

OCCUPATIONAL COMPETENCY EXAMINATIONS (OCE)

GENERAL

The Occupational Competency Examinations are intended for those individuals experienced in skilled trades or occupations who need to present objective evidence of their competency to become vocational teachers, to obtain academic credit from a higher institution, or to secure teacher certification.

In addition to meeting university admission requirements for fully matriculated students -- and for teacher certification -successful completion of the exam provides opportunity to earn up to 36 semester hours of collegiate credit for applied occupational skills and technical knowledge. The credit may be used toward advanced study and degrees in occupational education in several states.

NATURE OF THE EXAMINATION

The examination consists of two parts -- Written and Performance. The written test covers factual knowledge, technical information, understanding of principles and problem solving abilities related to the occupation. The performance test is designed to sample the manipulative skills required by an occupation. Thus it enables the candidate to demonstrate that he possesses the knowledge and skills that a competent craftsman employs in his daily work.

ADVANTAGES

The Prospective Teacher - Tradesmen and other technically competent persons who wish to enter industrial education training programs.

Industrial Teacher Educators - The OCE Tests provide the industrial teacher educator with an objective and dependable means for assessing the trade competency of applicants for admission to their programs.

Certifying Agencies - The OCE Tests provide an objective method for assessing occupational competence in qualifying for certification.

Directors of Vocational Education Programs - The OCE Tests provide a recruitment and selection procedure that is reliable, objective and fair to all recipients

Candidates for Academic Degrees - The OCE Tests are accepted by many colleges and universities for granting of credit or advanced standing for occupational experience.

PLACE OF EXAMINATION

A network of 36 Area Test Centers has been established throughout the United States in the States listed below. Tests are generally conducted twice a year at these centers, as well as other locations, depending on need.

Alabama	Kentucky	Oregon
Arkansas	Massachusetts	Pennsylvania
California	Michigan	South Dakota
Colorado	Missouri	Tennessee
Connecticut	Montana	Texas
Florida	Nebraska	Utah
Georgia	New Jersey	Vermont
Hawaii	New York	Virginia
Idaho	North Dakota	Washington
Illinois	Ohio	West Virginia
Iowa	Oklahoma	Wisconsin

OCE TESTS OFFERED

Interested candidates are alerted to the occupations listed below as scheduled for examination. Individuals should notify the NOCTI if they wish to be examined in an occupation not listed.

- Air Conditioning and Refrigeration
- Airframe or Power plant Mechanics
- Appliance Repair
- Architectural Drafting
- Auto Body Repair
- Automatic Heating
- Auto Mechanics
- Building Maintenance
- Cabinetmaking and Millwork
- Carpentry
- Commercial and Advertising Art
- Commercial Photography
- Cosmetology
- Data Processing
- Dental Assisting
- Diesel Engine Repair
- Dressmaking
- Electrical Installation
- Electronics Communication
- General Printing Industrial Electronics
- Machine Trades
- Masonry
- Machine Drafting
- Mechanical Technology
- Medical Assisting Offset Lithography
- Ornamental Horticulture
- Plumbing
- Quantity Food Preparation
- Sheet Metal Fabrication
- Small Engine Repair
- Welding

HOW TO REGISTER

For registration information contact Educational Testing Service of Princeton, New Jersey.

SCOPE FOR COSMETOLOGIST EXAMINATION

THE LICENSE EXAMINATION

The examination consists of <u>two parts</u>, a written part and practical part. Both parts are scheduled for the same day.
To pass the examination, you must achieve <u>all</u> of the following:

1. A score of at least 225 on the practical part
2. A score of at least 70 on the written part

If you pass both parts you will be issued a license immediately.
If you fail you will be given a form showing the scores in each category, the areas of failure, and an application form for re-examination with instructions.

SCOPE OF THE WRITTEN PART — 100 POINTS

SCIENTIFIC CONCEPTS 30%

Infection Control
- ◊ Microbiology
  - Bacteria
  - Viruses
  - Parasites
  - Immunity
  - Prevention
- ◊ Methods of infection control
  - Sanitation
  - Disinfection
  - Sterilization
- ◊ Federal regulations
  - OSHA guidelines
  - Material Safety Data Sheets (MSDS)
  - Environmental Protection Agency (EPA)
  - Food and Drug Administration (FDA)
  - Universal precautions
- ◊ First Aid
  - Minor bleeding
  - Minor burns
  - Minor eye irritation

Human Anatomy
- ◊ Cells
- ◊ Tissue
- ◊ Organs
  - Heart
  - Lungs
  - Skin

Basic Physiology (Body Systems)
- ◊ Skeletal system
  - Skull
  - Bones of the face
  - Bones of the neck
  - Bones of the shoulders
  - Bones of the arms and hands
  - Bones of the legs and feet
- ◊ Muscular system
  - Scalp muscles
  - Mastication muscles
  - Mouth muscles
  - Muscles of the eye and nose
  - Muscles of the arms and hands
  - Muscles of the legs and feet
  - Muscles of the neck
  - Muscles of the shoulders and upper back
- ◊ Types of joints
- ◊ Circulatory system
  - Blood-vascular or cardiovascular system
  - Lymph-vascular system
- ◊ Endocrine system
- ◊ Respiratory system
- ◊ Integumentary system
- ◊ Nervous system
- ◊ Excretory system

Ergonomics/Body Positioning

Basic Principles of Chemistry
- ◊ Matter
- ◊ The pH scale
- ◊ Nutrition
- ◊ Medication
- ◊ Compounds
- ◊ Mixtures
- ◊ Product ingredients
- ◊ Product labeling
- ◊ Product safety

Basic Principles of Electricity
- ◊ Electric current
- ◊ Electricity in cosmetology
  - Electrotherapy
  - Light therapy

HAIR CARE AND SERVICES 40%

Trichology
- ◊ Properties and structure of the hair and scalp
  - Shaft
  - Root
  - Keratinization
- ◊ Hair analysis and hair quality
  - Porosity
  - Elasticity
  - Texture
  - Density
- ◊ Stages of hair growth
- ◊ Hair loss
- ◊ Conditions of the scalp and hair
  - Disorders
  - Diseases

Draping Procedures
- ◊ Shampooing
- ◊ Haircutting
- ◊ Chemical services
- ◊ Thermal

Shampooing, Conditioning, Massaging and Brushing Procedures
- ◊ Hair analysis
- ◊ Scalp analysis
- ◊ Shampooing
  - Product selection
  - Procedure
- ◊ Conditioning
  - Product selection
  - Procedure
- ◊ Scalp treatments
- ◊ Scalp massage

Principles of Hair Design
- ◊ Elements of hair design
  - Form
  - Line/Direction
  - Growth pattern
  - Texture
  - Color
- ◊ Principles of balance and design
- ◊ Facial shapes

Haircutting Procedures
- ◊ Client consultation
  - Desired look
  - Face shape
  - Lifestyle and/or climate
  - Hair analysis
- ◊ Principles of haircutting
  - Areas of the head
  - Elevation or projection
  - Lines and angles
  - Crosschecking
  - Texturizing
- ◊ Tools and safety
  - Electrical
  - Manual
- ◊ Basic haircuts
  - Solid form or blunt haircut
  - Graduated form
  - Layered form
  - Combination form

Hairstyling Procedures
- ◊ Client consultation
- ◊ Wet styling
- ◊ Thermal styling
- ◊ Braiding

Wigs, Hair Enhancements and Extensions
- ◊ Client consultation
- ◊ Wigs and hair enhancements
  - Wig composition (e.g., human or synthetic)
  - Wig construction (e.g., cap and capless)

- Wig care
◊ Hair extensions and additions

Chemical Services Consultation
◊ Hair analysis
◊ Scalp analysis
◊ Predisposition (skin patch) test
◊ Preliminary strand test
◊ Desired results

Chemical Services
◊ Chemical waving
- pH balance of chemical waves
- Chemical waving procedures
◊ Chemical hair relaxers
- pH balance of chemical hair relaxers
- Chemical hair relaxing procedures

Haircoloring Procedures
◊ Law of color
◊ Types of haircolor
- Temporary haircolor
- Semi- and demi-permanent haircolor
- Permanent
- Lighteners
◊ Haircolor applications
- Virgin
- Retouch
- Color correction

SKIN CARE AND SERVICES 15%

Skin Histology
◊ Composition of the skin
- Layers of the skin
- Nerves of the skin
- Glands of the skin
- Types of skin
- Skin pigmentation
◊ Conditions of the skin
- Disorders
- Diseases
◊ Functions of the skin

Skin Care Services Consultation
◊ Skin analysis
◊ Health history

Draping Procedures for Facial Services

Temporary Hair Removal Procedures

◊ Shaving
◊ Tweezing
◊ Waxing
◊ Depilatories
◊ Threading
◊ Sugaring

Facial Procedures
◊ Skin care tools
- Equipment
- Implements
- Products and supplies
◊ Facial treatments
- Electrical therapy
- Massage manipulations
- Topical applications

Facial Makeup Application
◊ Makeup color theory
◊ Cosmetic application procedures
- Basic
- Specialty
- Corrective
◊ Artificial eyelashes
- Predisposition test
- Application
◊ Eyelash and eyebrow coloring

NAIL CARE AND SERVICES 15%

Nail Care Service Consultation

Nail Structure
◊ Nail composition
◊ Nail growth
◊ Nail conditions
- Disorders
- Diseases

Manicure and Pedicure Procedures
◊ Nail care tools
- Equipment
- Implements
- Products and supplies
◊ Types of manicures and pedicures
- Basic manicure and pedicure
- Specialty manicures and pedicures
◊ Massage procedures
- Hand and arm massage
- Foot and leg massage
◊ Infection control procedures for pedicure basin

Advanced Nail Care

◊ Preservice and postservice procedures
◊ Nail tips
◊ Nail wraps and overlays
- Acrylics
- Gels
◊ Nail art

SAMPLE QUESTIONS

The following sample questions are similar to those on the NIC Cosmetology Written Examination. Each question is followed by four answer choices. Only one choice is correct. Correct answers are listed following the sample questions.

1. Which of the following substances is usually contained in a toner?
   a. Metallic dye
   b. Compound dye
   c. Vegetable tint
   d. Oxidation tint

2. Which one of the following should be applied to the skin after removal of whiteheads?
   a. A caustic
   b. Deodorant
   c. An antiseptic
   d. Bleaching cream

3. Before disinfecting combs and brushes, they should be
   a. wiped with a towel.
   b. wiped with a tissue.
   c. rinsed in cold water.
   d. cleaned with soap and warm water.

4. What is the process used in tapering and thinning with scissors?
   a. Clipping
   b. Slithering
   c. Razor cutting
   d. Layer cutting

5. The action of chemical hair relaxers causes the hair to
   a. stop growing.
   b. harden and set.
   c. form new curls.
   d. soften and swell.

6. When should a predisposition test be performed?
   a. When the scalp has cuts
   b. Before applying peroxide
   c. Before every application of oxidizing tints
   d. Before any application of vegetable coloring

7. At what part of the nail does growth start?
   a. Wall
   b. Matrix
   c. Lunula
   d. Cuticle

8. What is the function of sebum?
   a. To dry the skin
   b. To harden the skin
   c. To cleanse the skin
   d. To lubricate the skin

9. Sterilization is the process of
   a. keeping bacteria alive.
   b. destroying offensive odors.
   c. destroying beneficial microorganisms only.
   d. destroying both harmful and beneficial bacteria.

10. Where should freshly laundered towels be kept?
    a. On a clean shelf
    b. In any convenient place
    c. In a closed cabinet or drawer
    d. In neat stacks by the shampoo bowl

Answers		
1. d	4. b	7. b 10. c
2. c	5. d	8. d
3. d	6. c	9. d

HOW TO TAKE A TEST

You have studied long, hard and conscientiously.

With your official admission card in hand, and your heart pounding, you have been admitted to the examination room.

You note that there are several hundred other applicants in the examination room waiting to take the same test.

They all appear to be equally well prepared.

You know that nothing but your best effort will suffice. The "moment of truth" is at hand: you now have to demonstrate objectively, in writing, your knowledge of content and your understanding of subject matter.

You are fighting the most important battle of your life—to pass and/or score high on an examination which will determine your career and provide the economic basis for your livelihood.

What extra, special things should you know and should you do in taking the examination?

I. YOU MUST PASS AN EXAMINATION

A. WHAT EVERY CANDIDATE SHOULD KNOW

Examination applicants often ask us for help in preparing for the written test. What can I study in advance? What kinds of questions will be asked? How will the test be given? How will the papers be graded?

B. HOW ARE EXAMS DEVELOPED?

Examinations are carefully written by trained technicians who are specialists in the field known as "psychological measurement," in consultation with recognized authorities in the field of work that the test will cover. These experts recommend the subject matter areas or skills to be tested; only those knowledges or skills important to your success on the job are included. The most reliable books and source materials available are used as references. Together, the experts and technicians judge the difficulty level of the questions.

Test technicians know how to phrase questions so that the problem is clearly stated. Their ethics do not permit "trick" or "catch" questions. Questions may have been tried out on sample groups, or subjected to statistical analysis, to determine their usefulness.

Written tests are often used in combination with performance tests, ratings of training and experience, and oral interviews. All of these measures combine to form the best-known means of finding the right person for the right job.

II. HOW TO PASS THE WRITTEN TEST

A. BASIC STEPS

1) Study the announcement

How, then, can you know what subjects to study? Our best answer is: "Learn as much as possible about the class of positions for which you've applied." The exam will test the knowledge, skills and abilities needed to do the work.

Your most valuable source of information about the position you want is the official exam announcement. This announcement lists the training and experience qualifications. Check these standards and apply only if you come reasonably close to meeting them. Many jurisdictions preview the written test in the exam announcement by including a section called "Knowledge and Abilities Required," "Scope of the Examination," or some similar heading. Here you will find out specifically what fields will be tested.

2) Choose appropriate study materials

If the position for which you are applying is technical or advanced, you will read more advanced, specialized material. If you are already familiar with the basic principles of your field, elementary textbooks would waste your time. Concentrate on advanced textbooks and technical periodicals. Think through the concepts and review difficult problems in your field.

These are all general sources. You can get more ideas on your own initiative, following these leads. For example, training manuals and publications of the government agency which employs workers in your field can be useful, particularly for technical and professional positions. A letter or visit to the government department involved may result in more specific study suggestions, and certainly will provide you with a more definite idea of the exact nature of the position you are seeking.

3) Study this book!

III. KINDS OF TESTS

Tests are used for purposes other than measuring knowledge and ability to perform specified duties. For some positions, it is equally important to test ability to make adjustments to new situations or to profit from training. In others, basic mental abilities not dependent on information are essential. Questions which test these things may not appear as pertinent to the duties of the position as those which test for knowledge and information. Yet they are often highly important parts of a fair examination. For very general questions, it is almost impossible to help you direct your study efforts. What we can do is to point out some of the more common of these general abilities needed in public service positions and describe some typical questions.

1) General information

Broad, general information has been found useful for predicting job success in some kinds of work. This is tested in a variety of ways, from vocabulary lists to questions about current events. Basic background in some field of work, such as sociology or economics, may be sampled in a group of questions. Often these are principles which have become familiar to most persons through exposure rather than through formal training. It is difficult to advise you how to study for these questions; being alert to the world around you is our best suggestion.

2) Verbal ability

An example of an ability needed in many positions is verbal or language ability. Verbal ability is, in brief, the ability to use and understand words. Vocabulary and grammar tests are typical measures of this ability. Reading comprehension or paragraph interpretation questions are common in many kinds of civil service tests. You are given a paragraph of written material and asked to find its central meaning.

IV. KINDS OF QUESTIONS

1. Multiple-choice Questions

Most popular of the short-answer questions is the "multiple choice" or "best answer" question. It can be used, for example, to test for factual knowledge, ability to solve problems or judgment in meeting situations found at work.

A multiple-choice question is normally one of three types:
- It can begin with an incomplete statement followed by several possible endings. You are to find the one ending which best completes the statement, although some of the others may not be entirely wrong.
- It can also be a complete statement in the form of a question which is answered by choosing one of the statements listed.
- It can be in the form of a problem – again you select the best answer.

Here is an example of a multiple-choice question with a discussion which should give you some clues as to the method for choosing the right answer:

When an employee has a complaint about his assignment, the action which will best help him overcome his difficulty is to
- A. discuss his difficulty with his coworkers
- B. take the problem to the head of the organization
- C. take the problem to the person who gave him the assignment
- D. say nothing to anyone about his complaint

In answering this question, you should study each of the choices to find which is best. Consider choice "A" – Certainly an employee may discuss his complaint with fellow employees, but no change or improvement can result, and the complaint remains unresolved. Choice "B" is a poor choice since the head of the organization probably does not know what assignment you have been given, and taking your problem to him is known as "going over the head" of the supervisor. The supervisor, or person who made the assignment, is the person who can clarify it or correct any injustice. Choice "C" is, therefore, correct. To say nothing, as in choice "D," is unwise. Supervisors have and interest in knowing the problems employees are facing, and the employee is seeking a solution to his problem.

2. True/False

3. Matching Questions

Matching an answer from a column of choices within another column.

V. RECORDING YOUR ANSWERS

Computer terminals are used more and more today for many different kinds of exams.

For an examination with very few applicants, you may be told to record your answers in the test booklet itself. Separate answer sheets are much more common. If this separate answer sheet is to be scored by machine – and this is often the case – it is highly important that you mark your answers correctly in order to get credit.

VI. BEFORE THE TEST

YOUR PHYSICAL CONDITION IS IMPORTANT

If you are not well, you can't do your best work on tests. If you are half asleep, you can't do your best either. Here are some tips:

1) Get about the same amount of sleep you usually get. Don't stay up all night before the test, either partying or worrying—DON'T DO IT!
2) If you wear glasses, be sure to wear them when you go to take the test. This goes for hearing aids, too.
3) If you have any physical problems that may keep you from doing your best, be sure to tell the person giving the test. If you are sick or in poor health, you relay cannot do your best on any test. You can always come back and take the test some other time.

Common sense will help you find procedures to follow to get ready for an examination. Too many of us, however, overlook these sensible measures. Indeed, nervousness and fatigue have been found to be the most serious reasons why applicants fail to do their best on civil service tests. Here is a list of reminders:

- Begin your preparation early – Don't wait until the last minute to go scurrying around for books and materials or to find out what the position is all about.
- Prepare continuously – An hour a night for a week is better than an all-night cram session. This has been definitely established. What is more, a night a week for a month will return better dividends than crowding your study into a shorter period of time.
- Locate the place of the exam – You have been sent a notice telling you when and where to report for the examination. If the location is in a different town or otherwise unfamiliar to you, it would be well to inquire the best route and learn something about the building.
- Relax the night before the test – Allow your mind to rest. Do not study at all that night. Plan some mild recreation or diversion; then go to bed early and get a good night's sleep.
- Get up early enough to make a leisurely trip to the place for the test – This way unforeseen events, traffic snarls, unfamiliar buildings, etc. will not upset you.
- Dress comfortably – A written test is not a fashion show. You will be known by number and not by name, so wear something comfortable.
- Leave excess paraphernalia at home – Shopping bags and odd bundles will get in your way. You need bring only the items mentioned in the official notice you received; usually everything you need is provided. Do not bring reference books to the exam. They will only confuse those last minutes and be taken away from you when in the test room.

- Arrive somewhat ahead of time – If because of transportation schedules you must get there very early, bring a newspaper or magazine to take your mind off yourself while waiting.
- Locate the examination room – When you have found the proper room, you will be directed to the seat or part of the room where you will sit. Sometimes you are given a sheet of instructions to read while you are waiting. Do not fill out any forms until you are told to do so; just read them and be prepared.
- Relax and prepare to listen to the instructions
- If you have any physical problem that may keep you from doing your best, be sure to tell the test administrator. If you are sick or in poor health, you really cannot do your best on the exam. You can come back and take the test some other time.

VII. AT THE TEST

The day of the test is here and you have the test booklet in your hand. The temptation to get going is very strong. Caution! There is more to success than knowing the right answers. You must know how to identify your papers and understand variations in the type of short-answer question used in this particular examination. Follow these suggestions for maximum results from your efforts:

1) Cooperate with the monitor

The test administrator has a duty to create a situation in which you can be as much at ease as possible. He will give instructions, tell you when to begin, check to see that you are marking your answer sheet correctly, and so on. He is not there to guard you, although he will see that your competitors do not take unfair advantage. He wants to help you do your best.

2) Listen to all instructions

Don't jump the gun! Wait until you understand all directions. In most civil service tests you get more time than you need to answer the questions. So don't be in a hurry. Read each word of instructions until you clearly understand the meaning. Study the examples, listen to all announcements and follow directions. Ask questions if you do not understand what to do.

3) Identify your papers

Civil service exams are usually identified by number only. You will be assigned a number; you must not put your name on your test papers. Be sure to copy your number correctly. Since more than one exam may be given, copy your exact examination title.

4) Plan your time

Unless you are told that a test is a "speed" or "rate of work" test, speed itself is usually not important. Time enough to answer all the questions will be provided, but this does not mean that you have all day. An overall time limit has been set. Divide the total time (in minutes) by the number of questions to determine the approximate time you have for each question.

5) Do not linger over difficult questions

If you come across a difficult question, mark it with a paper clip (useful to have along) and come back to it when you have been through the booklet. One caution if you do this – be sure to skip a number on your answer sheet as well. Check often to be sure that you have not lost your place and that you are marking in the row numbered the same as the question you are answering.

6) Read the questions

Be sure you know what the question asks! Many capable people are unsuccessful because they failed to read the questions correctly.

7) Answer all questions

Unless you have been instructed that a penalty will be deducted for incorrect answers, it is better to guess than to omit a question.

8) Speed tests

It is often better NOT to guess on speed tests. It has been found that on timed tests people are tempted to spend the last few seconds before time is called in marking answers at random – without even reading them – in the hope of picking up a few extra points. To discourage this practice, the instructions may warn you that your score will be "corrected" for guessing. That is, a penalty will be applied. The incorrect answers will be deducted from the correct ones, or some other penalty formula will be used.

9) Review your answers

If you finish before time is called, go back to the questions you guessed or omitted to give them further thought. Review other answers if you have time.

10) Return your test materials

If you are ready to leave before others have finished or time is called, take ALL your materials to the monitor and leave quietly. Never take any test material with you. The monitor can discover whose papers are not complete, and taking a test booklet may be grounds for disqualification.

VIII. EXAMINATION TECHNIQUES

1) Read the general instructions carefully. These are usually printed on the first page of the exam booklet. As a rule, these instructions refer to the timing of the examination; the fact that you should not start work until the signal and must stop work at a signal, etc. If there are any special instructions, such as a choice of questions to be answered, make sure that you note this instruction carefully.

2) When you are ready to start work on the examination, that is as soon as the signal has been given, read the instructions to each question booklet, underline any key words or phrases, such as least, best, outline, describe and the like. In this way you will tend to answer as requested rather than discover on reviewing your paper that you listed without describing, that you selected the worst choice rather than the best choice, etc.

3) If the examination is of the objective or multiple-choice type – that is, each question will also give a series of possible answers: A, B, C or D, and you are called upon to select the best answer and write the letter next to that answer on your answer paper – it is advisable to start answering each question in turn. There may be anywhere from 50 to 100 such questions in the three or four hours allotted and you can see how much time would be taken if you read through all the questions before beginning to answer any. Furthermore, if you

come across a question or group of questions which you know would be difficult to answer, it would undoubtedly affect your handling of all the other questions.

4) If the examination is of the essay type and contains but a few questions, it is a moot point as to whether you should read all the questions before starting to answer any one. Of course, if you are given a choice – say five out of seven and the like – then it is essential to read all the questions so you can eliminate the two that are most difficult. If, however, you are asked to answer all the questions, there may be danger in trying to answer the easiest one first because you may find that you will spend too much time on it. The best technique is to answer the first question, then proceed to the second, etc.

5) Time your answers. Before the exam begins, write down the time it started, then add the time allowed for the examination and write down the time it must be completed, then divide the time available somewhat as follows:
    - If 3-1/2 hours are allowed, that would be 210 minutes. If you have 80 objective-type questions, that would be an average of 2-1/2 minutes per question. Allow yourself no more than 2 minutes per question, or a total of 160 minutes, which will permit about 50 minutes to review.
    - If for the time allotment of 210 minutes there are 7 essay questions to answer, that would average about 30 minutes a question. Give yourself only 25 minutes per question so that you have about 35 minutes to review.

6) The most important instruction is to read each question and make sure you know what is wanted. The second most important instruction is to time yourself properly so that you answer every question. The third most important instruction is to answer every question. Guess if you have to but include something for each question. Remember that you will receive no credit for a blank and will probably receive some credit if you write something in answer to an essay question. If you guess a letter – say "B" for a multiple-choice question – you may have guessed right. If you leave a blank as an answer to a multiple-choice question, the examiners may respect your feelings but it will not add a point to your score. Some exams may penalize you for wrong answers, so in such cases only, you may not want to guess unless you have some basis for your answer.

7) Suggestions
    a. Objective-type questions
        1. Examine the question booklet for proper sequence of pages and questions
        2. Read all instructions carefully
        3. Skip any question which seems too difficult; return to it after all other questions have been answered
        4. Apportion your time properly; do not spend too much time on any single question or group of questions
        5. Note and underline key words – all, most, fewest, least, best, worst, same, opposite, etc.
        6. Pay particular attention to negatives
        7. Note unusual option, e.g., unduly long, short, complex, different or similar in content to the body of the question
        8. Observe the use of "hedging" words – probably, may, most likely, etc.

9. Make sure that your answer is put next to the same number as the question
10. Do not second-guess unless you have good reason to believe the second answer is definitely more correct
11. Cross out original answer if you decide another answer is more accurate; do not erase until you are ready to hand your paper in
12. Answer all questions; guess unless instructed otherwise
13. Leave time for review

b. Essay questions
1. Read each question carefully
2. Determine exactly what is wanted. Underline key words or phrases.
3. Decide on outline or paragraph answer
4. Include many different points and elements unless asked to develop any one or two points or elements
5. Show impartiality by giving pros and cons unless directed to select one side only
6. Make and write down any assumptions you find necessary to answer the questions
7. Watch your English, grammar, punctuation and choice of words
8. Time your answers; don't crowd material

8) Answering the essay question

Most essay questions can be answered by framing the specific response around several key words or ideas. Here are a few such key words or ideas:

M's: manpower, materials, methods, money, management
P's: purpose, program, policy, plan, procedure, practice, problems, pitfalls, personnel, public relations

a. Six basic steps in handling problems:
1. Preliminary plan and background development
2. Collect information, data and facts
3. Analyze and interpret information, data and facts
4. Analyze and develop solutions as well as make recommendations
5. Prepare report and sell recommendations
6. Install recommendations and follow up effectiveness

b. Pitfalls to avoid
1. Taking things for granted – A statement of the situation does not necessarily imply that each of the elements is necessarily true; for example, a complaint may be invalid and biased so that all that can be taken for granted is that a complaint has been registered
2. Considering only one side of a situation – Wherever possible, indicate several alternatives and then point out the reasons you selected the best one
3. Failing to indicate follow up – Whenever your answer indicates action on your part, make certain that you will take proper follow-up action to see how successful your recommendations, procedures or actions turn out to be
4. Taking too long in answering any single question – Remember to time your answers properly

EXAMINATION SECTION

EXAMINATION SECTION
TEST 1

DIRECTIONS: Each question or incomplete statement is followed by several suggested answers or completions. Select the one that *BEST* answers the question or completes the statement. *PRINT THE LETTER OF THE CORRECT ANSWER IN THE SPACE AT THE RIGHT.*

1. The coarseness or fineness of hair is determined by its
   A. porosity   B. diameter   C. melanin   D. elasticity

2. If the papilla is destroyed, then the hair will
   A. grow again   B. grow longer
   C. grow thinner   D. never grow again

3. Hair pigment is derived from the color-forming substances in the
   A. skin   B. liver   C. blood   D. lymph

4. Normal hair when wet, can be stretched *approximately*
   A. 50%   B. 20%   C. 75%   D. 40%

5. The cause of dry skin can be traced to a lack of
   A. pores   B. sebum   C. hormones   D. enzymes

6. The small openings of the sweat glands on the skin are called
   A. follicles   B. capillaries   C. pores   D. roots

7. The sebaceous glands of the skin secrete
   A. melanin   B. lymph   C. oil   D. perspiration

8. The skin is thickest on the
   A. palms and soles   B. ears
   C. eyebrows   D. face

9. A shaping which resembles the outline of a wave but which does not have a definite ridge and formation is called a _____ wave.
   A. skip   B. halo
   C. interlocking   D. shadow

10. To produce a good wave line, it is necessary that you have
    A. wavy hair   B. a planned pattern
    C. straight hair   D. a test curl

11. A pin curl placed immediately behind or below a ridge to form a wave is called a(n) _____ curl.

    A. cascade
    B. ridge
    C. upward
    D. reverse

12. A combination of a ridge against which is placed a series of overlapping pin curls followed by another ridge and series of pin curls is called a(n) _____ wave.

    A. halo
    B. skip
    C. interlocking
    D. vertical

13. The elevation or crest of a wave is known as the wave

    A. ridge   B. stem   C. spiral   D. crown

14. The diameter of the pin curl will determine the

    A. width of the wave
    B. depth of the wave
    C. direction of the ridge
    D. direction of the wave

15. The proper results in comb pressing will be retarded by the application of too much

    A. wrist movement
    B. pressing oil
    C. heat
    D. tension

16. The type of hair which usually requires the MOST heat in thermal waving is _____ hair.

    A. fine
    B. tinted
    C. false
    D. coarse

17. Fish hooks in thermal curling may be the direct result of forming _____ curls.

    A. incomplete
    B. tight
    C. overlapping
    D. loose

18. When forming a thermal curl, the iron is inserted at *approximately* a _____ - degree angle.

    A. 45
    B. 60
    C. 75
    D. 30

19. For the protection of the patron's scalp in thermal waving, the operator should

    A. dampen the hair roots
    B. hold a finger under the curl
    C. hold the hair up and away from the scalp
    D. click the iron frequently

20. A lightener retouch is applied to

    A. the entire hair shaft
    B. the hair ends
    C. the new growth of the hair
    D. a virgin head of hair

21. The process of adding artificial color to the hair is known as hair

    A. toning   B. tinting   C. oxidizing   D. lightening

22. White henna is a(n)

    A. powdered magnesium carbonate
    B. organic dye
    C. lightening agent
    D. oil bleach

23. Lightened hair requires special care because it may be

    A. less porous
    B. excessively oily
    C. excessively elastic
    D. dry and fragile

24. Hair breakage may result if a lighteneer is applied over hair previously treated with

    A. cholesterol
    B. sulphur ointment
    C. cream rinse
    D. a metallic hair dye

25. An aniline derivative hair dye is an example of

    A. compound henna
    B. penetrating hair tint
    C. vegetable hair tint
    D. metallic hair tint

KEY (CORRECT ANSWERS)

1.	B	11.	B
2.	D	12.	B
3.	C	13.	A
4.	D	14.	B
5.	B	15.	B
6.	C	16.	D
7.	C	17.	A
8.	A	18.	A
9.	D	19.	B
10.	B	20.	C

21. B
22. B
23. D
24. D
25. B

TEST 2

DIRECTIONS: Each question or incomplete statement is followed by several suggested answers or completions. Select the one that BEST answers the question or completes the statement. PRINT THE LETTER OF THE CORRECT ANSWER IN THE SPACE AT THE RIGHT.

1. The part of the hair which MOST readily absorbs the hair tint is the 1.____
   - A. side of the head
   - B. back of the head
   - C. hair ends
   - D. hair near the scalp

2. Facial massage is beneficial because it simultates the 2.____
   - A. salivary glands
   - B. pituitary glands
   - C. blood circulation
   - D. thyroid glands

3. Improper cleansing of the skin may cause the development of 3.____
   - A. blackheads
   - B. lentigo
   - C. furuncles
   - D. lesions

4. A clay pack is recommended for a skin that has 4.____
   - A. moles
   - B. warts
   - C. lesions
   - D. blackheads

5. Friction in massage requires the use of _____ movements. 5.____
   - A. pinching
   - B. slapping
   - C. deep stroking
   - D. light stroking

6. Effleurage is used in massage for _____ effects. 6.____
   - A. cooling
   - B. soothing and relaxing
   - C. heating
   - D. magnetic

7. A scalp that can be moved easily with finger manipulation is called _____ scalp. 7.____
   - A. loose
   - B. dry
   - C. free
   - D. galvanic

8. Hair pieces are BEST cleaned with a(n) _____ shampoo. 8.____
   - A. liquid dry
   - B. powder dry
   - C. soap
   - D. egg

9. Color rinses produce a _____ hair. 9.____
   - A. lighter shade to dark
   - B. temporary coloring to the
   - C. yellowish tinge in gray
   - D. permanent coloring to the

10. Soapless oil shampoo is composed of _____ oil. 10.____
    - A. sulfonated
    - B. crude
    - C. lanolin
    - D. mineral

11. A liquid dry shampoo may contain 11.____

    A. orris root
    B. henna mixture
    C. liquid soap
    D. a cleansing fluid

12. Waves are formed by 12.____

    A. half circles going in opposite directions
    B. half circles going in same direction
    C. two ridges directed to the right
    D. two ridges directed to the left

13. A wave shaped toward the face is called a 13.____

    A. French twist
    B. forward wave
    C. pompadour
    D. skip wave

14. The strand of hair from the scalp up to but not including the first curvature of the curl is called the 14.____

    A. hair cuticle
    B. curl ridge
    C. curl stem
    D. curl base

15. In setting hair, if the comb does NOT penetrate to the scalp, the wave will 15.____

    A. be more lasting
    B. not last
    C. be frizzy
    D. be deeper

16. The opening and blending of the hair setting, curls, waves, etc., into the finished coiffure is called a 16.____

    A. planned pattern
    B. natural growth pattern
    C. style setting
    D. comb-out

17. For a side part, the finger waving usually is started on the 17.____

    A. thin side of the hair
    B. back of the head
    C. heavy side of the hair
    D. crown of the head

18. Combing the short hairs toward the scalp is known as 18.____

    A. featheredging
    B. back combing
    C. effileing
    D. tipping

19. The BEST results in finger waving are obtained when the hair is 19.____

    A. straight
    B. naturally wavy
    C. frizzy
    D. kinky

20. To form pin curls that will be lasting and springy, it is necessary that the hair be wet, flat and 20.____

    A. very oily
    B. excessively curly
    C. away from the base
    D. stretched

21. In order that we form good pin curls, the hair must 21.____

    A. be slightly twisted
    B. have a natural wave
    C. be flat and smooth
    D. lie away from the base

22. The choice of setting lotion should be governed by 22.____

    A. its lightening qualities
    B. the color of the lotion
    C. the texture of the patron's hair
    D. its lacquer content

23. A good comb-out of a hair style is simplified by 23.____

    A. the use of a good setting lotion
    B. a planned hair-set
    C. combing hair slightly damp
    D. using curls with small center openings

24. In mixing the tint with the developer, use a _____ dish. 24.____

    A. brass   B. copper
    C. glass   D. bronze

25. A developer is an oxidizing agent such as 25.____

    A. ammonia   B. hydrogen peroxide
    C. dye softener   D. dye solvent

KEY (CORRECT ANSWERS)

1.	C	11.	D
2.	C	12.	A
3.	A	13.	B
4.	D	14.	C
5.	C	15.	B
6.	B	16.	D
7.	A	17.	C
8.	A	18.	B
9.	B	19.	B
10.	A	20.	D

21. C
22. C
23. B
24. C
25. B

EXAMINATION SECTION
TEST 1

DIRECTIONS: Each question or incomplete statement is followed by several suggested answers or completions. Select the one that *BEST* answers the question or completes the statement. *PRINT THE LETTER OF THE CORRECT ANSWER IN THE SPACE AT THE RIGHT.*

1. A chemical agent which will prevent the growth of germs is called a(n) 1.____
   - A. toxin
   - B. antiseptic
   - C. septic
   - D. astringent

2. Creams should be removed from jars with 2.____
   - A. the corner of a towel
   - B. a spatula
   - C. the fingers
   - D. a pledget

3. An agent which causes the contraction of living organic tissue and thus checks bleeding is called a(n) 3.____
   - A. antiseptic
   - B. disinfectant
   - C. styptic
   - D. glycerine

4. When not in use, sanitized instruments should be kept in 4.____
   - A. the pocket
   - B. a dry sanitizer
   - C. an insecticide
   - D. a deodorizer

5. Bacteria will be destroyed by 5.____
   - A. glycerine
   - B. intense heat
   - C. pumice
   - D. freezing

6. Bacteria can enter the body through 6.____
   - A. hair
   - B. nails
   - C. broken skin
   - D. unbroken skin

7. Instruments which *must* be sanitized regularly should be made of 7.____
   - A. brass
   - B. stainless steel
   - C. tin plated copper
   - D. aluminum

8. Pathogenic bacteria create 8.____
   - A. immunity
   - B. disease
   - C. anti-toxins
   - D. hormones

9. Milium is the technical name for a 9.____
   - A. whitehead
   - B. blackhead
   - C. pimple
   - D. dry skin

10. Pediculosis capitis is the technical term for 10.____
    - A. head lice
    - B. itch mites
    - C. flies
    - D. mosquitoes

11. Frequent washings with strong soaps may cause the scalp to become

    A. healthy   B. oily   C. dry   D. flexible

12. The hair and scalp may often be reconditioned with heating cap treatments and

    A. lemon rinses   B. porosity treatments
    C. scalp massage   D. stripping treatments

13. A tint to which peroxide has been added

    A. penetrates the hair shaft
    B. gives an orange tone to the hair
    C. coats the hair shaft
    D. lightens the hair

14. A temporary coating of color applied to the hair is called a

    A. compound dyestuff   B. metallic tint
    C. progressive tint   D. color rinse

15. A penetrating tint is one which penetrates and deposits color permanently into the

    A. cuticle   B. medulla   C. cortex   D. follicle

16. Hair containing no red or gold tones is known as _____ hair.

    A. drab   B. lightened
    C. brunette   D. tinted

17. Hair should NEVER be thinned close to the

    A. sides   B. crown   C. ends   D. scalp

18. The hair should be wet if hairshaping is done with

    A. shears   B. clippers
    C. razor   D. thinning scissors

19. Thinning the hair involves

    A. shortening   B. blunt cutting
    C. decreasing its bulk   D. trimming the ends

20. Removal of split hair ends may be accomplished by

    A. ruffing   B. slithering
    C. blunt cutting D. feathering

21. Featheredging the neckline is BEST accomplished with

    A. a coarse toothed comb   B. a lighted wax taper
    C. a razor   D. points of the shears

22. Shortening and thinning the hair at the same time is known as

    A. clipping   B. ruffing   C. tapering   D. back-combing

23. In basic hair shaping, the length of the strands of hair should NOT vary by more than 23.____
    A. 2 inches   B. 1/4 inch   C. 1 inch   D. 1 1/2 inches

24. Before hair is set, it is important that it be 24.____
    A. shaped   B. clipped   C. ruffed   D. shingled

25. The BEST time to apply scalp manipulations in shampooing is 25.____
    A. before the head has been lathered
    B. after the head has been lathered
    C. after the head has been rinsed
    D. after the head has been dried

KEY (CORRECT ANSWERS)

1. B	11. C
2. B	12. C
3. C	13. A
4. B	14. D
5. B	15. C
6. C	16. A
7. B	17. D
8. B	18. C
9. A	19. C
10. A	20. C

21. D
22. C
23. B
24. A
25. B

TEST 2

DIRECTIONS: Each question or incomplete statement is followed by several suggested answers or completions. Select the one that BEST answers the question or completes the statement. PRINT THE LETTER OF THE CORRECT ANSWER IN THE SPACE AT THE RIGHT.

1. When shampooing lightened hair, use

    A. a mild shampoo and tepid water
    B. hot water
    C. liquid dry shampoo
    D. strong shampoo

    1.____

2. When pressing hair over a loose scalp, use

    A. large sections   B. more oil
    C. small sections   D. more pressure

    2.____

3. The EASIEST type of hair to press is _____ hair.

    A. coarse   B. wiry
    C. fine   D. gray

    3.____

4. The PROPER position to hold a strand of hair while it is being wound is to hold it

    A. in a downward position
    B. to one side
    C. up and out from the scalp
    D. in a slanting position

    4.____

5. Cold wave curls are wrapped without tension to

    A. give a loose wave
    B. give a tight wave
    C. allow the hair to contract
    D. prevent overprocessing

    5.____

6. The neutralizing time in cold permanent waving is comparable to one of the following in heat permanent waving:

    A. steaming time   B. cooling time
    C. wrapping time   D. test curl time

    6.____

7. In giving a cold wave to tinted hair, you must expect

    A. the true hair shade to appear   B. some discoloration
    C. the hair to become darker   D. some hair breakage

    7.____

8. Cold wave solution applied to the scalp may cause scalp

    A. discoloration   B. irritation   C. tension   D. wens

    8.____

9. End papers used in winding hair ends for a cold permanent wave must be

    A. non-porous   B. moisture proof
    C. porous   D. dampened with a fixative

    9.____

10. If tension is used in winding the hair, the action of the cold wave solution may be

    A. retarded
    B. accelerated
    C. stopped entirely
    D. neutralized

11. The deciding factor in determining the processing time in cold permanent waving is the hair

    A. texture   B. pigment   C. porosity   D. density

12. Sectioning and winding the hair for a cold permanent wave usually begins at the _____ area.

    A. crown
    B. frontal
    C. nape
    D. temple

13. Before starting a cold permanent wave, the hair should be shampooed and thoroughly

    A. lubricated
    B. saturated
    C. rinsed
    D. neutralized

14. A cosmetology license issued by the division of licenses is *not* needed for an operator who gives only

    A. shampoos
    B. scalp treatments
    C. manicures
    D. facials

15. The texture of hair that requires the LONGEST processing time in cold permanent waving is _____ hair.

    A. fine   B. wiry   C. bleached   D. dyed

16. A preparation used in beauty culture that is *highly* inflammable is

    A. brilliantine
    B. astringent
    C. hair lacquer
    D. cold-wave lotion

17. A bluing rinse may be given

    A. to tone down over-hennaed hair
    B. to give a platinum shade to bleached hair
    C. to take the yellow out of gray or white hair
    D. for all the above purposes

18. Upon entering a beauty shop, you find that the operator, in preparation for a patron, has assembled, gauze, orris powder, shaker, hair tonic, cotton, hair brush. You would surmise that the preparation is for a

    A. scalp treatment for oily hair
    B. scalp treatment for dry hair
    C. pre-shampoo treatment
    D. dry shampoo

19. Comb pressing is known as a _____ press.

    A. regular   B. marcel   C. hard   D. soft

20. A substance that is NOT present in hair is   20.____

    A. carbon   B. hydrogen   C. nitrogen   D. kaoline

21. Of the following, the MOST recent development in correcting broken and bitten nails is   21.____
the application of

    A. "Nail Fix"   B. "Patti Nails"
    C. artificial nails   D. Revlon's "Lactol"

22. Electrolysis permanently removes hair by destroying the hair   22.____

    A. shaft   B. root   C. bulb   D. papilla

23. The purpose of the neutralizer in the cold-wave process is to   23.____

    A. fix the curl   B. expand the hair
    C. soften the hair   D. remove the oil from the hair

24. Which of the following statements is INCORRECT?   24.____

    A. A knowledge of hair porosity is important to a beauty operator who does hair tinting.
    B. The ends of the hair take tint slower than the rest of the hair
    C. 28% ammonia water is used in some bleaching mixtures.
    D. Powdered magnesium carbonate is sometimes used when bleaching hair with hydrogen peroxide and ammonia water.

25. Which of the following statements is INCORRECT?   25.____

    A. Metallic hair tints are recommended by professional beauticians.
    B. It is sometimes necessary to pre-soften hair in giving a hair tint.
    C. A beautician should know when it is advisable to use a hair filler
    D. Under proper conditions bleached hair can usually be given a successful permanent wave.

KEY (CORRECT ANSWERS)

1. A
2. C
3. A
4. D
5. C

6. B
7. B
8. B
9. C
10. A

11. A
12. C
13. B
14. C
15. B

16. C
17. D
18. D
19. D
20. D

21. B
22. D
23. A
24. B
25. A

EXAMINATION SECTION
TEST 1

DIRECTIONS: Each question or incomplete statement is followed by several suggested answers or completions. Select the one that BEST answers the question or completes the statement. PRINT THE LETTER OF THE CORRECT ANSWER IN THE SPACE AT THE RIGHT.

1. A substance having the ability to check the growth and multiplication of bacteria without destroying them, is called a(n)   1._____

   A. germicide   B. deodorant   C. antiseptic   D. disinfectant

2. A disinfectant can be applied with safety to   2._____

   A. the body   B. instruments
   C. clothing   D. an opening in the skin

3. Pathogenic bacteria are   3._____

   A. beneficial   B. harmful
   C. harmless   D. not disease producing

4. Asteatosis is an   4._____

   A. abundance of the sebaceous secretions
   B. absence of the sebaceous secretions
   C. abundance of the sudoriferous secretions
   D. absence of the sudoriferous secretions

5. A vinegar rinse is a(n) _____ rinse.   5._____

   A. alkaline   B. neutral
   C. acid   D. coloring

6. A dry shampoo is given with   6._____

   A. liquid soap   B. powdered orris root
   C. powdered soap   D. an antiseptic

7. The study of the nervous system and its disorders is called   7._____

   A. myology   B. dermatology   C. histology   D. neurology

8. The dead cells of the stratum corneum   8._____

   A. never shed   B. constantly flake off
   C. shed according to season   D. are difficult to remove

9. The skin is an absorbing organ to   9._____

   A. a limited extent   B. a great extent
   C. no extent   D. liquids only

10. Inflammation of the skin is known as

    A. dermatology B. dermatosis
    C. dermatologist D. dermatitis

11. Astringent tonics or ointments are most effective on

    A. normal skin B. dry skin
    C. oily skin D. sunburned skin

12. The use of strong soaps should be avoided on _____ skin.

    A. oily B. normal
    C. freckled D. dry

13. Face powders are intended to improve the _____ of the skin.

    A. texture B. appearance
    C. color D. function

14. Dry, brittle nails are aggravated by

    A. hot oil treatments B. tissue cream
    C. alkaline soaps D. cuticle cream

15. A group of similar cells performing the same function is called a(n)

    A. organ B. tissue C. gland D. system

16. In cleaning the free edge of the nail, abrasions are less likely to occur if the operator uses a(n)

    A. metal cleaner B. small brush
    C. orangewood stick D. bone instrument

17. The harmless types of hair colorings are the

    A. metallic dyes B. vegetable dyes
    C. aniline dyes D. compound hennas

18. The medical term for gray hair is

    A. albinism B. canities C. leucoderma D. lentigo

19. The addition of a few drops of a 28% solution of ammonia to peroxide will

    A. hasten its bleaching action
    B. stop its bleaching action
    C. lessen its bleaching action
    D. make the bleach more lasting

20. The treatment for trichoptilosis is

    A. thinning B. shingling C. clipping D. bobbing

21. Located at the back and lower part of the cranium is the

    A. frontal bone B. occipital bone
    C. parietal bone D. temporal bone

22. In machine permanent waving, coarse hair requires 22.____
    A. the same steaming time as fine hair
    B. less steaming time than fine hair
    C. more steaming time than fine hair
    D. double the steaming time for fine hair

23. The technical name for baldness is 23.____
    A. alopecia   B. pityriasis   C. dermatitis   D. albinism

24. Scalp treatments are NOT intended to 24.____
    A. preserve the health of the hair
    B. correct dandruff or loss of hair
    C. stimulate glandular activity
    D. cure infectious diseases of the scalp and hair

25. Processing in cold waving should be determined by 25.____
    A. the amount of hair   B. test curl
    C. texture of hair   D. previous waving time

KEY (CORRECT ANSWERS)

1.	C	11.	C
2.	B	12.	D
3.	B	13.	B
4.	B	14.	C
5.	C	15.	B
6.	B	16.	C
7.	D	17.	B
8.	B	18.	B
9.	A	19.	A
10.	D	20.	C

21. B
22. B
23. A
24. D
25. C

TEST 2

DIRECTIONS: Each question or incomplete statement is followed by several suggested answers or completions. Select the one that BEST answers the question or completes the statement. PRINT THE LETTER OF THE CORRECT ANSWER IN THE SPACE AT THE RIGHT.

1. It is advisable to brush hair before giving a shampoo because it   1.____
   A. saves combing after shampoo
   B. stimulates the scalp
   C. helps the operator to give the shampoo more rapidly
   D. saves one soaping

2. When bacteria get into the body, they are usually destroyed by   2.____
   A. white blood cells   B. red blood cells
   C. lymph   D. plasma

3. Nails are composed of keratin, which is also found in the   3.____
   A. muscles   B. hair shaft   C. glands   D. bones

4. Eyelashes should NOT be tinted with hair dye because   4.____
   A. it may cause injury to the eyes
   B. it may not match the hair
   C. it may be too strong and make them too dark
   D. the operator may not be experienced in using it

5. Overbleached hair is difficult to permanent-wave because it has lost its   5.____
   A. melanin   B. elasticity   C. medulla   D. cortex

6. A spiral flat wave is   6.____
   A. twisted   B. half-twisted
   C. wound from ends to roots   D. wound from roots to ends

7. Excessive perspiration may be caused by   7.____
   A. cold   B. mental excitement
   C. lack of exercise   D. relaxation

8. A condition in which the cuticle splits around the nail is known as   8.____
   A. felon   B. onychia   C. hangnail   D. infection

9. A comedone extractor is a small instrument for removing   9.____
   A. scars   B. pimples   C. milia   D. blackheads

10. Nails are composed of a horny protein substance called   10.____
    A. cortex   B. keratin   C. allergens   D. cicatrix

11. The amount of melanin in the hair determines the   11.____
    A. texture   B. strength   C. elasticity   D. color

18

12. A disinfectant can also be used as an antiseptic if it is

    A. diluted
    B. concentrated
    C. applied full strength in smaller quantity
    D. mixed with a germicide

13. Hair is more resistant to dye

    A. behind the ears
    B. at the back of the head
    C. at the crown
    D. at the forehead and temples

14. A license which entitles an operator to work in a city beauty shop is issued by the

    A. department of health
    B. department of state
    C. department of labor
    D. city bureau of licenses

15. If, during the manicure, the skin is cut, the operator should apply

    A. powdered alum
    B. formalin
    C. styptic pencil
    D. herpicide

16. Pediculosis is treated by the application of

    A. tincture of larkspur
    B. oil of wintergreen
    C. lanolin
    D. vinegar

17. To disentangle oversteamed hair, one should use a(n)

    A. alkaline rinse
    B. peroxide rinse
    C. neutral rinse
    D. acid rinse

18. Of the following, the harmless types of hair colorings are the

    A. aniline dyes
    B. compound henna
    C. metallic dyes
    D. vegetable dyes

19. Which of these statements about bone is untrue?

    A. The technical term for bone is os.
    B. Bone is composed of animal and mineral matter.
    C. Bone is pink externally and white internally.
    D. The two types of bone tissue are dense and cancellous.

20. Which of these statements is untrue?

    A. Boiling water destroys all bacteria except spores.
    B. Spore-forming bacteria can be destroyed by exposure to steam at 15 pounds pressure.
    C. Dry heat is often used in the beauty shop.
    D. A disinfectant solution can be changed to an antiseptic by dilution.

21. Chemicals should be stored in

    A. open containers in a dark, dry and cool place
    B. closed containers in a dark, dry and cool place
    C. closed containers in a light, damp and cool place
    D. closed containers in a dark, damp and warm place

22. How should coarse hair and fine hair be wound for cold-waving? 22.____

    A. Coarse hair should be wound in smaller curls than fine hair.
    B. Coarse hair should be wound in larger curls than fine hair.
    C. Coarse hair cannot be cold-waved as easily as fine hair.
    D. Coarse hair takes a shorter time than fine hair for cold-waving.

23. Which of these statements is untrue? The 23.____

    A. ends of the bones are covered with cartilage
    B. occipital bone is located at the crown
    C. cranium consists of 10 bones
    D. mandible bone is bone of the lower jaw

24. Ringworm on the skin is caused by a 24.____

    A. bacterium   B. fungus   C. protozoan   D. worm

25. Cold applications tend to 25.____

    A. decrease the supply of blood in the area to which they are applied
    B. dilate the blood vessels
    C. bring a greater supply of blood to the area to which they are applied
    D. increase the pressure on the nerve endings

KEY (CORRECT ANSWERS)

1.	B	11.	D
2.	A	12.	A
3.	B	13.	C
4.	A	14.	B
5.	B	15.	A
6.	D	16.	A
7.	B	17.	D
8.	C	18.	D
9.	D	19.	C
10.	B	20.	C

21. B
22. A
23. B
24. B
25. A

EXAMINATION SECTION
TEST 1

DIRECTIONS: Each question or incomplete statement is followed by several suggested answers or completions. Select the one that BEST answers the question or completes the statement. PRINT THE LETTER OF THE CORRECT ANSWER IN THE SPACE AT THE RIGHT.

1. Which of the following statements are CORRECT?   1.____
    - I. The skin is the same thickness over the entire body.
    - II. Hair is an appendage of the nails.
    - III. Keratin is the horny substance of which hair is made.
    - IV. The amount of pigment contained in the cortex determines the color of hair.

   The CORRECT answer is:

   A. I, II B. I, III C. III, IV D. II, IV

2. Which of the following statements is (are) CORRECT?   2.____
    - I. Keratosis is a form of skin disease characterized by thinning epidermis.
    - II. An acute disease is one of long duration.
    - III. Canities is caused by fever, shock, nervousness, or senility.
    - IV. Eczema is a contagious, parasitic disease of the skin, with crust formations, emitting a mousy odor.

   The CORRECT answer is:

   A. III only B. I only C. II, III D. III, IV

3. Which of the following statements is (are) INCORRECT?   3.____
    - I. Lanolin is a beneficial ingredient in tissue creams.
    - II. The eyes should be covered with pads when exposing the face to therapeutic lights.
    - III. Muscle toning treatments are recommended for oily skin.
    - IV. Massage helps to eliminate the waste products of metabolism.

   The CORRECT answer is:

   A. III only B. IV only C. I, II D. III, IV

4. Which of the following statements is (are) INCORRECT?   4.____
    - I. A dry shampoo cleanses the hair by absorbing the dirt and oil.
    - II. Cocoanut oil is a desirable ingredient in shampoos because it helps to form a thick lather.
    - III. A gasoline shampoo is dangerous because it is inflammable.
    - IV. Vinegar and lemon rinses help to neutralize the alkaline soap residue on the hair and scalp.

   The CORRECT answer is:

   A. I only   B. I, II, III
   C. I, II, III, IV   D. None of the above

5. Which of the following statements is (are) CORRECT?
    I. The most hygienic way to stimulate the circulation of the scalp is by scratching it.
    II. In the treatment for alopecia, the high-frequency current is applied with a glass rake electrode but without sparks.
    III. The cosmetologist is most concerned with the treatment of scalp diseases.
    IV. A shampoo rarely accompanies a scalp treatment.
    The CORRECT answer is:

    A. I only   B. II only   C. I, III, IV   D. II, III

6. Which of the following statements is (are) INCORRECT?
    I. Ordinary household ammonia can be used to mix with peroxide for bleaching purposes.
    II. The newer growth near the scalp is most resistant to a hair dye.
    III. It is better to be lavish than sparing in the use of hair tint.
    IV. A synthetic hair dye is progressive in action; whereas a hair color restorer acts instantaneously.
    The CORRECT answer is:

    A. II only   B. I, II, III   C. II, III, IV   D. I, III, IV

7. Which of the following statements is (are) INCORRECT?
    I. Pointed neck lines are suggested for long, slender necks.
    II. The principal difference between a shingle bob and a feather-edge is the height at which the hair is cut.
    III. The thumb is uppermost on the scissors when shingling or feather-edging.
    IV. In singeing the hair, the lighted taper is passed over loose hair.
    The CORRECT answer is:

    A. II only   B. I, II, III   C. II, III, IV   D. I, III, IV

8. Which of the following statements are CORRECT?
    I. It is better to oversteam than to understeam the hair.
    II. It is always advisable to make a test curl.
    III. Hair of a porous nature is the most difficult to wave.
    IV. A vinegar rinse will help to remove snarls occasioned by oversteamed or kinky hair.
    The CORRECT answer is:

    A. I, II   B. I, III   C. III, IV   D. II, IV

9. Which of the following statements are INCORRECT?
    I. Recommend beauty treatments which offer the greatest profits, without considering the benefits to the patron.
    II. A spiral permanent wave can be substituted for a croquignole permanent wave.
    III. Trade practices and secrets can be revealed to the public.
    IV. An operator is justified in condemning her competitors.
    The CORRECT answer is:

    A. I, II, III, IV   B. I, II, III
    C. II, III, IV   D. I, III, IV

10. Which of the following statements are CORRECT? 10.____
    I. The skin is the organ of protection, absorption, elimination, heat regulation, respiration, and sensation.
    II. Age has no effect on the elasticity of the skin.
    III. The skin is the seat of the organ of touch.
    IV. The sebaceous glands secrete an oily substance called sebum.

The CORRECT answer is:

A. I, II, III
C. I, III, IV
B. II, III, IV
D. I, II, IV

KEY (CORRECT ANSWERS)

1. C
2. A
3. A
4. D
5. B

6. D
7. D
8. D
9. A
10. C

TEST 2

DIRECTIONS: Each question or incomplete statement is followed by several suggested answers or completions. Select the one that *BEST* answers the question or completes the statement. *PRINT THE LETTER OF THE CORRECT ANSWER IN THE SPACE AT THE RIGHT.*

1. Which of the following statements is (are) *CORRECT*?
    I. Keloid is a wartlike growth commonly located in the eyelids.
    II. A communicable disease is one that can be transmitted from person to person.
    III. Alopecia areata is baldness at time of birth.
    IV. Pityriasis is the term applied to an excessively oily condition of the scalp.
    The *CORRECT* answer is:

    A. I, II, III B. II, III, IV C. III, IV D. II *only*

    1.____

2. Which of the following statements is (are) *CORRECT*?
    I. Fine skin requires less cleansing treatments than coarse skin.
    II. Astringent lotion lubricates the underlying tissues.
    III. Makeup of all kinds should correspond to the natural coloring of the individual.
    IV. Cleansing creams are absorbed by the skin.
    The *CORRECT* answer is:

    A. III *only* B. II, III C. I, III D. IV *only*

    2.____

3. Which of the following statements is (are) *INCORRECT*?
    I. Corns should be removed when giving a pedicure.
    II. Alcohol is a good remedy for perspiring hands.
    III. Hydrogen peroxide solution is used as a germicide in manicuring.
    IV. The nail blade has a vascular supply while the matrix has none.
    The *CORRECT* answer is:

    A. II *only* B. I, II, III C. II, III, IV D. I, III, IV

    3.____

4. Which of the following statements is (are) *INCORRECT*?
    I. A peroxide rinse is used to give the hair a reddish tint.
    II. Henna rinse and henna compound have the same base.
    III. Tar shampoos are advised for light hair only.
    IV. Egg shampoos are advised for bleached, dry and brittle hair.
    The *CORRECT* answer is:

    A. I, II B. I *only* C. III, IV D. I, III

    4.____

5. Which of the following statements is (are) *CORRECT*?
    I. Synthetic organic dyes are penetrating dyes.
    II. Metallic dyes only coat the hair shaft.
    III. Any person can receive a hair dye with perfect safety.
    IV. A predisposition test is only applied if a lesion or an inflammation of the scalp is present.
    The *CORRECT* answer is:

    A. I, II, III B. II, III, IV C. I *only* D. I, II

    5.____

6. Which of the following statements is (are) INCORRECT?
    I. A correct haircut will emphasize the attractive features and minimize the defects.
    II. Alcohol may be used for sterilizing clippers and shears.
    III. Bangs are best suited to a face with a high forehead.
    IV. The hair should be thinned before a marcel wave.
    The CORRECT answer is:

    A. I, II   B. II, III   C. I, II, IV   D. III only

7. Which of the following statements are CORRECT?
    I. Medium warm irons are employed for croquignole marcel waving.
    II. Start a croquignole marcel wave at the back of the head.
    III. In marcelling, the hair should be picked up with a comb, not with an iron.
    IV. Brushing and combing injure marcel waves.
    The CORRECT answer is:

    A. I, II   B. II, III   C. III, IV   D. I, IV

8. Which of the following statements is (are) INCORRECT?
    I. All systems of heat permanents are dependent upon moisture, alkali, contraction and expansion of the hair.
    II. Average healthy hair can be stretched about twenty percent of its own length.
    III. The hydroscopic quality of hair means its ability to absorb liquids.
    IV. When hair becomes too kinky from a permanent wave, hot oil treatments will help.
    The CORRECT answer is:

    A. I, II, III, IV   B. I, II, III
    C. II, III   D. None of the above

9. Which of the following statements is (are) CORRECT?
    I. An operator can discuss controversial issues in a beauty shop.
    II. The borrowing and lending of supplies and instruments are to be encouraged.
    III. Do not represent a marcel wave to be the same as a finger wave.
    IV. Inferior supplies can be substituted for standard goods.
    The CORRECT answer is:

    A. I, II, IV   B. I, II   C. III only   D. II, III, IV

10. Which of the following statements are INCORRECT?
    I. The appendages of the skin are the nails, hair, sebaceous and sudoriferous glands.
    II. Skin absorbs water readily.
    III. Health, age, and occupation have no influence on the texture of the skin.
    IV. Elimination is an important function of the skin.
    The CORRECT answer is:

    A. I, II   B. II, III   C. III, IV   D. I, IV

KEY (CORRECT ANSWERS)

1. D
2. A
3. D
4. D
5. D

6. D
7. B
8. D
9. C
10. B

COSMETOLOGY
EXAMINATION SECTION
TEST 1

DIRECTIONS: Each question or incomplete statement is followed by several suggested answers or completions. Select the one that *BEST* answers the question or completes the statement. *PRINT THE LETTER OF THE CORRECT ANSWER IN THE SPACE AT THE RIGHT.*

1. Which of the following statements are INCORRECT?
    I. Hot packs are recommended for acne rosacea treatments.
    II. Dandruff is considered a disease if the shedding of scales is excessive.
    III. An albino is a person with an abnormal deficiency of pigment in the skin, hair, and eyes.
    IV. Oily foods tend to aggravate a dry condition of the skin.
   The answer is:

   A. I, II, III   B. I, III, IV   C. I, IV   D. II, IV

   1.____

2. Which of the following statements are CORRECT?
    I. Skin bleaching lubricates the skin.
    II. Heat causes the skin to contract.
    III. Facials may be given once a week if necessary.
    IV. Vanishing creams are non-absorbent and serve as a powder base.
   The answer is:

   A. I, II   B. II, III   C. III, IV   D. II, IV

   2.____

3. Which of the following statements are INCORRECT?
    I. The shape of the nail is determined by the shape of the finger.
    II. The nail should be filed from the center to the corners.
    III. Hangnails are a splitting of the epidermis at the side of the finger.
    IV. Liquid polish is injurious to the nail.
   The answer is:

   A. II, IV   B. II, III   C. I, III   D. I, IV

   3.____

4. Which of the following statements is (are) CORRECT?
    I. Yellow streaks in white hair may be caused by acid in the system.
    II. Water that is too hot dries the scalp.
    III. Water is composed of hydrogen and oxygen.
    IV. Heated oil is not good for general use on the hair.
   The answer is:

   A. IV *only*   B. I, II, III   C. I, II, IV   D. II, III, IV

   4.____

5. Which of the following statements is (are) INCORRECT?
    I. Ammonia added to a bleach always gives a reddish tint.
    II. Tinting of hair has been practiced in recent years only.
    III. When changing the color of the hair which has a uniform color, it is necessary to dye first that portion which was last treated with the softener.
    IV. White henna is a bleach.
   The answer is:

   A. III *only*   B. I, II, III   C. I, II, IV   D. II, III, IV

   5.____

6. Which of the following statements are CORRECT?
    I. The treatment for trichoptilosis is clipping or singeing.
    II. A number one hair clipper makes the shortest cut.
    III. A good hair comb is made of hard rubber.
    IV. Use a fresh neck strip and towel for each customer.
    The answer is:

    A. I, II, III, IV
    B. I, II, III
    C. I, III, IV
    D. II, III, IV

7. Which of the following statements are INCORRECT?
    I. Marcelling cannot be accomplished with kinky hair.
    II. It is not necessary to stretch the hair in order to produce a lasting wave.
    III. It is necessary to use a hot iron on bleached hair.
    IV. The temperature of the irons should not be the same for every texture of hair.
    The answer is:

    A. I, II, III
    B. I, II, IV
    C. I, III, IV
    D. II, III, IV

8. Which of the following statements are CORRECT?
    I. Always start a finger wave at the back of the head.
    II. Finger waving is easier to accomplish if the proper waving lotion is used.
    III. The hair should be thoroughly combed before finger waving.
    IV. After the finger wave is formed, it is not necessary to reset waves into a soft coiffure.
    The answer is:

    A. I, II
    B. I, III
    C. II, III
    D. III, IV

9. Which of the following statements are INCORRECT?
    I. A successful permanent wave can be given over a hair restorer.
    II. In a croquignole permanent wave, the protectors are attached to the head before the hair is wound.
    III. There is no difference between a wet and dry winding since both are treated with pads.
    IV. A spiral permanent wave is usually wound from the hair ends to the scalp.
    The answer is:

    A. I, II, III
    B. II, III, IV
    C. I, III, IV
    D. I, II, IV

10. Which of the following statements are CORRECT?
    I. Operators should accept tips.
    II. The operator should not try to sell the patron additional services while giving her a facial.
    III. The operator can discuss personal matters while giving a beauty treatment.
    IV. Promptness in keeping appointments helps to retain patrons.
    The answer is:

    A. I, III
    B. II, III
    C. I, IV
    D. II, IV

KEY (CORRECT ANSWERS)

1. C
2. C
3. A
4. B
5. C

6. C
7. A
8. C
9. C
10. D

TEST 2

DIRECTIONS: Each question or incomplete statement is followed by several suggested answers or completions. Select the one that BEST answers the question or completes the statement. *PRINT THE LETTER OF THE CORRECT ANSWER IN THE SPACE AT THE RIGHT.*

1. Which of the following statements are INCORRECT?
    I. Corium, derma, and true skin are the same.
    II. The skin is an external non-flexible covering of the body.
    III. Dermatology is the study of the hair.
    IV. The skin is an organ of elimination.
   The answer is:

   A. I, III   B. II, III   C. I, IV   D. II, IV

2. Which of the following statements is (are) CORRECT?
    I. Pityriasis is the presence of white scales in the hair and scalp.
    II. Pityriasis is the technical name for dandruff.
    III. The symptoms of pityriasis capitis are itching scalp, dry dandruff and a partial loss of hair.
    IV. Certain ingredients in cosmetics may cause a dermatitis.
   The answer is:

   A. I only   B. I, II   C. I, II, III   D. I, II, III, IV

3. Which of the following statements are INCORRECT?
    I. Tissue cream is used to nourish the skin.
    II. A double chin is due to a lack of adipose tissue.
    III. All eyebrows should be arched the same way.
    IV. Petrissage is a kneading movement.
   The answer is:

   A. I, II   B. II, III   C. II, IV   D. III, IV

4. Which of the following statements are CORRECT?
    I. Onychophagy should be treated as a disease.
    II. Nails filed long and given oil manicures will aid in keeping them from splitting.
    III. Onychia is inflammation of the nail matrix.
    IV. If a nail is torn, cut or injured, a new one will always grow.
   The answer is:

   A. I, II   B. II, III   C. II, IV   D. III, IV

5. Which of the following statements are INCORRECT?
    I. Always stimulate the scalp before each shampoo.
    II. Sage tea is a bleach.
    III. A vinegar rinse will cause hair to snarl.
    IV. An egg shampoo is recommended for overbleached hair.
   The answer is:

   A. I, II   B. II, III   C. II, IV   D. III, IV

6. Which of the following statements is (are) CORRECT?
    I. Hair can be dyed from a darker to a lighter shade.
    II. Ten-volume peroxide may be used just as effectively in bleaching hair as seventeen-volume.
    III. Hair may be tinted a lighter shade than the natural shade by just applying a lighter shade of tint.
    IV. Progressive dyes are slow working dyes.
   The answer is:

   A. I only   B. IV only   C. I, II, III   D. I, II, IV

7. Which of the following statements is (are) INCORRECT?
    I. A razor is never used for tapering and thinning.
    II. Neck dusters are never sterilized.
    III. It is advisable to singe the hair before shampooing.
    IV. Hair is always shampooed before cutting.
   The answer is:

   A. III only   B. IV only   C. I, II, III   D. I, II, IV

8. Which of the following statements are CORRECT?
    I. Round curls give a fluffy effect to fine, thin hair.
    II. Marcel waves should never be brushed.
    III. A hot iron should never be used when marcelling gray hair.
    IV. A Francois marcel and croquignole marcel are given in the same way.
   The answer is:

   A. I, II   B. II, III   C. I, III   D. II, IV

9. Which of the following statements are INCORRECT?
    I. Fine hair has more elasticity than coarse hair.
    II. Dyed hair should be steamed longer than normal hair.
    III. A full twist will give a marcel effect while a flat wrap will give a round curl effect on a spiral wrap permanent.
    IV. The steaming time on fine and coarse hair is the same, provided the wrap is different.
   The answer is:

   A. I, II   B. II, III   C. I, II, III   D. I, II, III, IV

10. Which of the following statements are CORRECT?
    I. Elasticity of hair is weakened by bleaching.
    II. Oversteamed hair can be restored to its original texture.
    III. All bleached hair can be given a successful permanent wave.
    IV. The width of the wave depends upon the amount of hair used in each strand.
   The answer is:

   A. I, II   B. I, III   C. I, IV   D. I, II, IV

KEYS (CORRECT ANSWERS)

1. B
2. D
3. B
4. B
5. B

6. B
7. D
8. C
9. D
10. C

EXAMINATION SECTION
TEST 1

DIRECTIONS: Each question or incomplete statement is followed by several suggested answers or completions. Select the one that BEST answers the question or completes the statement. *PRINT THE LETTER OF THE CORRECT ANSWER IN THE SPACE AT THE RIGHT.*

1. One way of inducing active immunity is to inject
    A. horse serum
    B. hormones
    C. streptomycin
    D. a vaccine

2. Pus usually contains bacteria plus
    A. fungi
    B. scar tissue
    C. red blood cells
    D. white blood cells

3. Among the major barriers to infection in the body are
    A. red blood cells
    B. striated muscle cells
    C. intestinal enzymes
    D. lymph nodes

4. Salk polio vaccine consists of
    A. living virus
    B. killed virus
    C. virus plus antibodies
    D. virus plus sulfa drugs

5. Pasteurization of milk
    A. destroys Vitamin C
    B. kills spore-forming bacteria
    C. is equivalent to sterilization
    D. involves boiling followed by cooling

6. Botulism, a serious form of food poisoning, is MOST often due to
    A. unsatisfactory home canning
    B. undercooking of meat
    C. exposure of food to flies
    D. exposure of food to air

7. All of the following foods may, if carelessly prepared, give rise to tapeworm infection EXCEPT
    A. beef
    B. fish
    C. fowl
    D. pork

8. Carriers are an important factor in the spread of
    A. diphtheria
    B. pellagra
    C. smallpox
    D. beri beri

9. Amebic dysentery may be prevented by the effective use of
    A. antibiotics
    B. immunization
    C. sewage disposal plants
    D. water chlorination

10. Of the following diseases, the one transmitted by insects is
    A. influenza
    B. trichinosis
    C. pneumonia
    D. typhus

11. The _____ is NOT part of the brain.   11.____
    A. medulla   B. cerebrum   C. meristem   D. all of the above

12. A cell is made up of   12.____
    A. fiber   B. protoplasm   C. nuclei   D. cytoplasm

13. A cell is   13.____
    A. made of tissues
    B. the smallest living unit in the body
    C. the largest living unit in the body
    D. found only in the extremities

14. Organs are composed of   14.____
    A. bi-unitary cells   B. singular cells
    C. tissue   D. groupings of tissue

15. Red blood cells are made in the   15.____
    A. red marrow of your bones   B. pancreas
    C. bloodstream   D. white marrow of your bones

16. All cells get their material for their growth and repair from   16.____
    A. foods   B. the same food
    C. minerals   D. H_2O

17. A material essential to protoplasm is   17.____
    A. protein   B. carbohydrate
    C. fat   D. sugar and starch

18. As cell structures differ, so   18.____
    A. do the connective tissues   B. does cell composition
    C. does the energy level   D. does the oxygen required

19. Carbohydrates, proteins, fats, minerals, vitamins, and water are all   19.____
    A. cells   B. energy   C. chemicals   D. nutrients

20. Scurvy can be prevented by   20.____
    A. vitamin C   B. ascorbic acid
    C. green vegetables   D. all of the above

21. A thermometer placed in your mouth for two minutes should NORMALLY read   21.____
    A. 96.6   B. 98.6   C. 98.7   D. 96.8

22. White blood cells   22.____
    A. are not necessary for life   B. are all white
    C. counteract bacteria   D. aid in digestion

23. The process of breaking down complex foods into simpler substances is called   23.____
    A. ingestion   B. acidation   C. digestion   D. absorption

24. The heart pumps blood into the aorta. This is a(n)
    A. vein   B. artery   C. capillary   D. artery capillary

25. An INCORRECT statement about the heart is that it
    A. is made of thick muscle   B. pumps blood
    C. never stops   D. all are correct

26. Bright red blood can MOST likely be found in
    A. veins   B. arteries
    C. vein capillaries   D. all of the above

27. The kidney
    A. stores fatty foods   B. creates bile
    C. removes waste from the blood   D. stores proteins

28. Bacteria
    A. can thrive without food
    B. live and feed on other organisms
    C. are never seen
    D. all of the above

29. Bacteria can be
    A. helpful   B. protected against
    C. overcome   D. all of the above

30. Penicillin is made from
    A. mold   B. blue cheese
    C. cows' milk   D. roots of a penicillin tree

31. The rod-shaped bacteria are called
    A. cocci   B. spirilla   C. bacilli   D. viruses

32. A germ killer that is made by a living organism is called a(n)
    A. inoculation   B. toxin   C. antibiotic   D. streptococci

33. Vaccination or inoculation causes the human body to
    A. building antibodies   B. build toxins
    C. get well   D. have natural immunity

34. The part of the cell that controls all the functions of the cell is the
    A. nucleus   B. endoplasm   C. cytoplasm   D. cell membrane

35. _____ is an element.
    A. Steel   B. Brass   C. Copper   D. Bronze

KEY (CORRECT ANSWERS)

1.	D	11.	C	21.	B	31.	C
2.	D	12.	B	22.	C	32.	C
3.	D	13.	B	23.	C	33.	A
4.	B	14.	D	24.	B	34.	A
5.	A	15.	A	25.	D	35.	C
6.	A	16.	A	26.	B		
7.	C	17.	A	27.	C		
8.	A	18.	B	28.	B		
9.	C	19.	D	29.	D		
10.	D	20.	D	30.	A		

TEST 2

DIRECTIONS: Each question or incomplete statement is followed by several suggested answers or completions. Select the one that BEST answers the question or completes the statement. *PRINT THE LETTER OF THE CORRECT ANSWER IN THE SPACE AT THE RIGHT.*

1. In the human body, ciliated cells are found in the
    A. blood vessels
    B. small intestine
    C. lining of the trachea
    D. lining of the kidney tubules

    1.____

2. In the human digestive system, enzymes are produced for the digestion of all of the following EXCEPT
    A. cane sugar
    B. corn starch
    C. cellulose
    D. vegetable oils

    2.____

3. In the developing human embryo, respiration takes place through the
    A. gills
    B. nostrils
    C. lungs
    D. placenta

    3.____

4. In the human embryo, the nervous system develops from the
    A. inner cell layer
    B. middle cell layer
    C. outer cell layer
    D. mesoderm

    4.____

5. The part of the eye affected in astigmatism is the
    A. cornea
    B. lens
    C. retina
    D. vitreous humor

    5.____

6. Dandruff is CHIEFLY composed of
    A. secretions of sebaceous glands
    B. dead epidermal cells
    C. yeast-like microbial organisms
    D. connective tissue from the scalp

    6.____

7. The white matter of the brain is made of
    A. nerve cell bodies
    B. axons and dendrites
    C. epithelial cells
    D. fat cells

    7.____

8. The behavior of a newborn child is characterized CHIEFLY by
    A. conditioned responses
    B. habit
    C. reflexes
    D. trial and error learning

    8.____

9. The organ that CANNOT be removed from the human body without causing death is
    A. the stomach
    B. the liver
    C. one kidney
    D. one lung

    9.____

10. A sphincter is a
    A. muscle that controls an opening
    B. joint of the ball-and-socket type
    C. gland producing both enzymes and hormones
    D. mass of nerve cells outside the spinal cord

11. The function of the parathyroid glands is to
    A. control calcium balance
    B. assure proper ovarian functions
    C. promote the digestion of starch
    D. aid in iron metabolism

12. The amount of blood in the body of an average man is normally _____ quarts.
    A. three   B. five   C. eight   D. ten

13. Red blood cells in the adult human being are formed in the
    A. bone marrow   B. liver
    C. lymph glands   D. heart

14. An artery containing blood relatively POOR in oxygen is the
    A. aorta   B. inferior vena cava
    C. superior vena cava   D. pulmonary

15. In tracer experiments designed to determine the length of life of red blood cells in the human body, the material used is an isotope of
    A. deuterium   B. gold   C. iron   D. phosphorus

16. A factor that is NOT necessary for the clotting of blood is
    A. prothrombin   B. air   C. calcium   D. fibrinogen

17. The structure that prevents food from passing into the windpipe is the
    A. esophagus   B. epiglottis   C. trachea   D. uvula

18. The HARDEST substance in the body is
    A. bone   B. cartilage   C. dentine   D. tooth enamel

19. The wrappings of the brain and spinal cord are
    A. epithelial tissues   B. meninges
    C. smooth muscles   D. striated muscles

20. The semicircular canals are PRIMARILY concerned with
    A. circulation of lymph   B. balance
    C. excretion   D. reproduction

21. Air pressure on both sides of the ear drum is equalized by the
    A. cochlea   B. ear bones
    C. Eustachian tubes   D. pharynx

3 (#2)

22. Memory is dependent upon the function of the 22.____
    A. cerebral cortex   B. cerebellum
    C. medulla   D. spinal cord

23. The amount of light entering the eye is regulated by the 23.____
    A. cornea   B. iris   C. retina   D. sclerotic coat

24. An inherited characteristic of man controlled by more than one pair of 24.____
    genes is
    A. hemophilia   B. red-green color blindness
    C. blood type   D. brown or blue eye color

25. The epidermis of the skin 25.____
    A. contains numerous capillaries
    B. contains the coiled portions of sweat glands
    C. includes some living cells
    D. is where the hair roots are located

KEY (CORRECT ANSWERS)

1.	C	11.	A
2.	C	12.	B
3.	D	13.	A
4.	C	14.	D
5.	A	15.	C
6.	B	16.	B
7.	B	17.	B
8.	C	18.	D
9.	B	19.	B
10.	A	20.	B

21. C
22. A
23. B
24. C
25. C

TEST 3

DIRECTIONS: Each question or incomplete statement is followed by several suggested answers or completions. Select the one that BEST answers the question or completes the statement. *PRINT THE LETTER OF THE CORRECT ANSWER IN THE SPACE AT THE RIGHT.*

1. The daily energy requirement in calories recommended by the National Academy of Sciences for the average high school girl is
   A. 1300 – 1500   B. 2400 – 2600   C. 3000 – 3200   D. 4800 - 5000

   1.____

2. The recommended dietary protein allowance for an individual is LEAST influenced by the factor of
   A. sex
   B. age
   C. type of activity
   D. weight

   2.____

3. Of the following diseases, the one which is NOT food-borne is
   A. diphtheria
   B. pneumonia
   C. tuberculosis
   D. scarlet fever

   3.____

4. Of the following, the disease which is caused by an agent in a different group from the agents causing the other three diseases is
   A. tobacco mosaic disease
   B. typhus
   C. measles
   D. polio

   4.____

5. Of the following, the one which is a HIGHLY contagious skin condition is
   A. eczema
   B. hives
   C. impetigo
   D. miliaria rubra

   5.____

6. Of the following, the antibiotic that has been found MOST effective in the treatment of tuberculosis is
   A. penicillin
   B. aureomycin
   C. streptomycin
   D. tetracycline

   6.____

7. Toxic effects in children have resulted from the ingestion of excessive amounts of which one of the following?
   A. Vitamin A
   B. Vitamin B_{12}
   C. Vitamin C
   D. Thiamine

   7.____

8. The basal metabolism test is ordinarily used to indicate
   A. hypertension
   B. activity of the thymus gland
   C. activity of the thyroid gland
   D. rate of blood circulation

   8.____

9. When Vitamin B_{12} is administered by mouth, it is of little or no value unless
   A. it is part of the Vitamin B complex
   B. normal gastric juice is present
   C. it has been extracted from liver
   D. it is taken in capsule form

   9.____

10. The *morale vitamin*, the lack of which may cause people to become depressed and irritable, is
    A. ascorbic acid   B. thiamine   C. riboflavin   D. folic acid

11. Of the following, the tissue that lines the hair follicle is called
    A. dermis   B. epidermis   C. adipose   D. subcutaneous

12. Microscopic examination of the cross-section of hair shafts of people with straight hair shows the hair shafts to be
    A. square   B. flat   C. round   D. oval

13. The outer layer of the hair shaft is called the
    A. cortex   B. medulla   C. cuticle   D. papilla

14. Grain alcohol is converted into acetic acid by which one of the following processes?
    A. Oxidation   B. Reduction   C. Methylation   D. Esterification

15. Dark spots occurring in canned foods are often caused by
    A. reaction of tannin in the food and iron in the can
    B. overcooking the food
    C. oxidation of the tin coating of the can
    D. use of hard water in canning

16. Undercooked poultry may cause
    A. tularemia   B. brucellosis
    C. salmonella poisoning   D. trichinosis

17. Certain diseases must be reported to the Department of Health Which one of the following is NOT required to be reported?
    A. Pneumonia
    B. Food poisoning occurring in a group of three or more cases
    C. Meningitis
    D. Trichinosis

18. Food charts indicate the amount of Vitamin A in foods in terms of
    A. grams   B. International Units
    C. milligrams   D. micrograms

19. A hormone which is secreted by the adrenal glands and which equips animals to prepare for emergencies is
    A. insulin   B. epinephrine
    C. thyroxin   D. progesterone

20. In humans, maintenance of constant body temperature is a prime function of the
    A. endocrines   B. skin
    C. muscles   D. excretory system

21. At which one of the following sites does fertilization in humans USUALLY occur?
    A. Fallopian tube
    B. Graafian follicle
    C. Ovary
    D. Uterus

22. The pulse beat felt at the wrist is the immediate result of
    A. systolic pressure
    B. heart beat
    C. venous response to heart beat
    D. arterial pressure changes felt on the wall of the artery

23. Glycogen is stored in
    A. bone and cartilage
    B. fatty tissue
    C. liver and muscle
    D. small intestine

24. A drug discovered in clover hay that is used to prevent blood clotting is
    A. chloromycetin
    B. dicoumarin
    C. digitalis
    D. meprobamate

25. Which one of the following tissues has the GREATEST amount of intercellular matrix?
    A. Visceral muscle
    B. Connective tissue
    C. Nerve tissue
    D. Epithelium

KEY (CORRECT ANSWERS)

1.	B		11.	B
2.	C		12.	C
3.	C		13.	D
4.	D		14.	C
5.	C		15.	A
6.	C		16.	C
7.	A		17.	A
8.	C		18.	B
9.	B		19.	B
10.	A		20.	B

21. A
22. D
23. C
24. B
25. B

EXAMINATION SECTION
TEST 1

DIRECTIONS: Each question or incomplete statement is followed by several suggested answers or completions. Select the one that BEST answers the question or completes the statement. *PRINT THE LETTER OF THE CORRECT ANSWER IN THE SPACE AT THE RIGHT.*

1. Forensic trichology can determine the _____ of the hair's owner.   1._____

   A. age
   B. body mass
   C. race
   D. all of the above

2. The only living portion of the hair is found in the hair   2._____

   A. follicle
   B. filament
   C. gland
   D. cuticle

3. What type of pigment is dominant in natural red hair?   3._____

   A. eumelanin
   B. pheomelanin
   C. exomelanin
   D. endomelanin

4. All of the following are characteristics of hair quality EXCEPT   4._____

   A. porosity
   B. texture
   C. elasticity
   D. rhythm

5. Hair grows everywhere on the body EXCEPT the   5._____

   A. soles of the feet
   B. lips
   C. palms of the hands
   D. all of the above

6. The anagen phase of hair growth can last up to   6._____

   A. 6 months
   B. 1 year
   C. 5 years
   D. 8 years

7. Sebum is a(n) _____ substance secreted by the sebaceous glands. 7._____

A. liquid
B. oily
C. granular
D. low viscosity

8. Trichotillomania is a disorder characterized by a(n) 8._____

A. normal amount of hair loss
B. compulsive urge to pull one's own hair
C. sexually transmitted disease
D. infection of the hair shaft

9. Male pattern baldness is also called 9._____

A. telogen effluvium
B. alopecia areata
C. androgenic alopecia
D. cicotricial alopecia

10. All of the following are treatments for hair loss EXCEPT 10._____

A. laser
B. hair plugs
C. minoxidil
D. rubbing compound

11. Which of the following is NOT a disorder of the scalp? 11._____

A. dandruff
B. tinea
C. nevus
D. scabies

12. *Pediculosis capitis* is also known as 12._____

A. dry scalp
B. dandruff
C. lice
D. psoriasis

13. When washing hair that has had a keratin treatment, always use a shampoo that is 13._____

A. for color-treated hair
B. for straight hair
C. sulfate-free
D. moisturizing

14. Hair is more fragile in all of the following circumstances EXCEPT when it is   14._____

A. natural
B. wet
C. flat-ironed
D. bleached

15. To avoid breakage, if hair is curly it should not be   15._____

A. brushed
B. combed when wet
C. shampooed daily
D. diffused

16. With regard to cutting hair, the term "angles" refers to the direction of the   16._____

A. scissors
B. razor
C. bottle
D. comb

17. When crosschecking a clipper cut, you would hold the comb   17._____

A. vertically
B. horizontally
C. diagonally
D. flat

18. Which of the following is a safety precaution for using a hairdryer?   18._____

A. Always unplug it after use
B. Do not use while bathing
C. Do not place in water
D. All of the above

19. Which of the following tools is NOT used to trim hair?   19._____

A. Shears
B. Razors
C. Clippers
D. Brush

20. Damaged hair is characterized by all of the following EXCEPT that   20._____

A. it has a rough texture
B. it is elastic
C. its color fades quickly
D. it is porous

4 (#1)

21. If a woman has thinning hair she may want   21._____

A. extensions
B. a wig
C. a hairpiece
D. all of the above

22. All of the following are types of permanent waves EXCEPT   22._____

A. alkaline
B. acid
C. dry
D. exothermic

23. Ammonium thioglycolate is an agent of   23._____

A. permanent waves
B. chemical relaxers
C. straightening products
D. conditioners

24. All of the following are types of chemical hair relaxers EXCEPT   24._____

A. alkaline
B. base
C. endothermic
D. no lye

25. The Fischer-Saller scale is to determine the _____ of human   25._____
hair.

A. thickness
B. shades
C. texture
D. length

KEY (CORRECT ANSWERS)

1. D	6. D	11. C	16. A	21. D
2. A	7. B	12. C	17. B	22. A
3. B	8. B	13. C	18. D	23. A
4. D	9. C	14. A	19. D	24. C
5. D	10. D	15. A	20. B	25. B

TEST 2

DIRECTIONS: Each question or incomplete statement is followed by several suggested answers or completions. Select the one that BEST answers the question or completes the statement. *PRINT THE LETTER OF THE CORRECT ANSWER IN THE SPACE AT THE RIGHT.*

1. Which of the following natural products can be used to lighten hair?   1._____

 A. lemon juice
 B. chamomile
 C. vinegar
 D. all of the above

2. Of the following chemicals, which is least damaging to the hair?   2._____

 A. Ammonia
 B. Citric acid
 C. Thioglycolic acid
 D. Hydrogen peroxide

3. What is used to open hair fiber so that dye molecules can settle in?   3._____

 A. Hydrogen peroxide
 B. Lead acetate
 C. Ammonia
 D. Acetone

4. A celebrity famous for his gray hair is   4._____

 A. Mario Lopez
 B. Richard Gere
 C. Antonio Banderas
 D. Brad Pitt

5. All of the following are common reasons to color hair EXCEPT to   5._____

 A. cover gray hair
 B. change to a color that is more fashionable or desirable
 C. restore the original color after it has been discolored
 D. do so accidentally

6. *Achromotrichia* is   6._____

 A. the process whereby hair turns gray or white as people age
 B. a disorder characterized by pulling one's own hair
 C. a disease of the scalp characterized by flaking skin
 D. the loss of hair from the body, including the scalp

7. Black hair is more common among 7._____

A. men than women
B. women than men
C. whites than non-white Hispanics
D. people from Europe than people from Japan

8. *Albinism* is 8._____

A. a genetic abnormality in which little or no pigment is found in the hair, eyes or skin
B. a patchy loss of hair and skin color that may occur as the result of an auto-immune disease
C. malnutrition causing the hair to become lighter, thinner and more brittle
D. a disorder characterized by premature aging

9. All of the following are common classifications for hair color EXCEPT 9._____

A. permanent
B. semi-permanent
C. demi-permanent
D. auto-permanent

10. All of the following techniques can be used to highlight hair EXCEPT 10._____

A. foiling, where pieces of foil or plastic film are used to separate off the hair to be colored
B. blanketing, with application to the hair as one overall color
C. balayage, where hair color is painted directly onto sections of the hair with no foils used to keep the color contained
D. cap, when a plastic cap is placed tight on the head and strands are pulled through with a hook

11. Special effects hair coloring refers to hair color 11._____

A. designed to create hair colors not typically found in nature
B. causing hair to become especially dark
C. which also makes hair more manageable
D. which also makes hair shiny

12. The best way to handle damaged hair is to 12._____

A. shampoo it everyday
B. deep condition it regularly
C. stop the use of chemicals until new hair grows and the damaged hair is cut off
D. both B and C

13. Lead acetate may

A. be toxic if ingested
B. cause stroke
C. affect blood flow
D. none of the above

14. Dyeing bleached hair brown can result in _____ hair.

A. slightly blue
B. gray or very ashy
C. lighter
D. very shiny

15. The primary colors are

A. red, blue and yellow
B. red, blue and green
C. orange, blue and yellow
D. white, gray and black

16. The possible adverse affects of hair coloring include all of the following EXCEPT

A. skin irritation and allergy
B. hair breakage
C. fingernail breakage
D. skin discoloration

17. Glaze is a liquid substance that is applied to _____ hair.

A. dry
B. wet
C. oily
D. dark

18. The hair's primary source of mechanical strength and water uptake is the

A. medulla
B. cuticle
C. cortex
D. follicle

19. The diameter of human hair varies from ____ to ____ µm.

A. 1; 10
B. 5; 25
C. 17; 180
D. 20; 105

20. If more melanin is present, the hair will appear   20._____

A. darker
B. lighter
C. thicker
D. thinner

21. Pheomelanin colors hair   21._____

A. blonde
B. red
C. brown
D. black

22. About _____ percent of people in the world have red hair.   22._____

A. 1 to 2
B. 5 to 10
C. 6 to 8
D. 10 to 15

23. Tobacco smoking can cause   23._____

A. hair darkening
B. premature graying
C. hair strengthening
D hair breakage

24. To remove semi-permanent hair color, shampoo containing _____ may be used.   24._____

A. lead acetate
B. sodium laurel sulfate
C. formaldehyde
D. chlorine

25. Symptoms of hair dye allergies include all of the following EXCEPT   25._____

A. skin inflammation
B. swelling or redness of the face
C. yellowing of the skin
D. difficulty breathing

KEY (CORRECT ANSWERS)

1. D	6. A	11. A	16. C	21. B
2. B	7. B	12. D	17. B	22. A
3. C	8. A	13. A	18. C	23. B
4. B	9. D	14. B	19. C	24. B
5. D	10. B	15. A	20. A	25. C

ANATOMY & PHYSIOLOGY
EXAMINATION SECTION
TEST 1

DIRECTIONS: Each question consists of a statement. You are to indicate whether the statement is TRUE (T) or FALSE (F). *PRINT THE LETTER OF THE CORRECT ANSWER IN THE SPACE AT THE RIGHT.*

1. A cell is a minute mass of protoplasm containing a nucleus. 1._____
2. Protoplasm is a jelly-like substance, present in all living matter. 2._____
3. Protoplasm is a lifeless matter. 3._____
4. Connective tissue serves to unite, support, and bind together other tissues. 4._____
5. Tendon is one of the varieties of connective tissue. 5._____
6. Muscle tissue is composed of cells modified to form fibers. 6._____
7. Organs are groups of systems. 7._____
8. Anabolism is the chemical change which involves the breaking down process within the cells. 8._____
9. Catabolism is the chemical change which involves the building up process within the cells. 9._____
10. Metabolism is the chemical change which involves the building up and breaking down process within the cells. 10._____
11. Nerves can be both motor and sensory. 11._____
12. Nerves can be stimulated by chemicals, massage, electricity, and heat. 12._____
13. Heat causes contraction of nerves. 13._____
14. Nervous fatigue is more prostrating than physical fatigue. 14._____
15. The cerebrum is the chief portion of the brain. 15._____
16. Nerves which carry information as to heat, cold, pressure, touch, and pain are called sensory nerves. 16._____
17. Sensory nerves and efferent nerves are the same. 17._____
18. The nervous system consists of cerebrospinal nervous system and the sympathetic nervous system. 18._____
19. The medulla oblongata is the bony structure protecting the brain. 19._____
20. Ganglia is a disease of the nervous system. 20._____

21. Nerves are a system of communication to all parts of the body. 21.___
22. Nerves have their origin in the brain. 22.___
23. Motor nerves carry impulses to the brain. 23.___
24. There are thirty-one pairs of cranial nerves. 24.___
25. There are fifteen pairs of spinal nerves. 25.___
26. The trifacial nerve is the smallest of all the cranial nerves. 26.___
27. The facial nerve is both motor and sensory. 27.___
28. The optic nerve is the nerve of the special sense of smell. 28.___
29. The mental nerve supplies lower lip and chin. 29.___
30. The temporal nerve supplies the frontalis muscle. 30.___
31. Mandibular nerve supplies the muscles of mastication. 31.___
32. The seventh pair of cranial nerves and the trifacial are the same. 32.___
33. The facial nerve supplies the muscles of expression in the face. 33.___
34. The lesser occipital nerve is a motor nerve. 34.___
35. The temporal is both sensory and motor nerve. 35.___
36. The blood vascular system controls the circulation of blood. 36.___
37. The walls of the arteries are elastic. 37.___
38. The veins lie deeper than the arteries. 38.___
39. General circulation is also known as systemic circulation. 39.___
40. Capillaries have thinner walls than arteries and veins. 40.___
41. About one-twentieth of the body weight is blood. 41.___
42. The heart is called an involuntary muscle. 42.___
43. Hemoglobin is the coloring matter of the red corpuscles. 43.___
44. Systemic circulation carries the blood from the heart to the lungs. 44.___
45. The blood carries oxygen to the cells and carbon dioxide from them. 45.___
46. Arteries carry the impure blood. 46.___
47. Study of the vascular system includes blood and lymph. 47.___
48. Red corpuscles attack germs that enter the blood. 48.___

49. Arteries, veins, and capillaries are tubular vessels. 49.____

50. A leucocyte is a red corpuscle. 50.____

51. Leucocyte is the technical term for white blood corpuscle. 51.____

52. Cardiac is the technical term for heart. 52.____

53. Circulation may be stimulated by physical and chemical means. 53.____

54. Lymph reaches parts of the body not reached by the blood. 54.____

55. The occipital artery supplies the forehead. 55.____

KEY (CORRECT ANSWERS)

1. T	11. T	21. T	31. T	41. T	51. T
2. T	12. T	22. T	32. F	42. T	52. T
3. F	13. F	23. F	33. T	43. T	53. T
4. T	14. T	24. F	34. F	44. F	54. T
5. T	15. T	25. F	35. T	45. T	55. F
6. T	16. T	26. F	36. T	46. F	
7. F	17. F	27. T	37. T	47. T	
8. F	18. T	28. F	38. F	48. F	
9. F	19. F	29. T	39. T	49. T	
10. T	20. F	30. F	40. T	50. F	

TEST 2

DIRECTIONS: Each question consists of a statement. You are to indicate whether the statement is TRUE (T) or FALSE (F). *PRINT THE LETTER OF THE CORRECT ANSWER IN THE SPACE AT THE RIGHT.*

1. The technical term for bone is os. 1.____
2. Bone is composed of animal and mineral matter. 2.____
3. Bone is pink externally and white internally. 3.____
4. The external membrane covering bone is called pericardium. 4.____
5. The shafts of long bones are solid. 5.____
6. The two types of bone tissue are dense and cancellous. 6.____
7. Dense tissue forms the interior of bone and cancellous tissue the exterior of bone. 7.____
8. The cranium is the bony case which encases the brain. 8.____
9. The skull is the technical term given the skeleton of the head. 9.____
10. The skull includes the cranial and the facial bones. 10.____
11. Red and white corpuscles are derived from red and yellow bone marrow. 11.____
12. Articulations and joints are the same. 12.____
13. Periosteum is a disease of the bone. 13.____
14. The entire skeleton consists of 106 bones. 14.____
15. The ends of bones are covered with cartilage. 15.____
16. The occipital bone is located at the crown. 16.____
17. The parietal bones are located at the forehead. 17.____
18. Maxillae are bones which form the upper jaw. 18.____
19. The cranium consists of ten bones. 19.____
20. The ethmoid is a small bone of the ear. 20.____
21. The malar bones form the prominence of the cheeks. 21.____
22. The turbinal bones form the eyesockets. 22.____
23. The mandible is the bone of the lower jaw. 23.____
24. The frontal bone forms the cheeks. 24.____
25. The temporal bones are located in the ear region. 25.____

26. Cartilage is sometimes called gristle.   26._____
27. Muscles are the active organs of locomotion.   27._____
28. The heart muscles are described as non-striated.   28._____
29. Voluntary muscles are controlled by the will.   29._____
30. The cardiac is a voluntary muscle.   30._____
31. Aponeurosis is a fibrous membrane.   31._____
32. Muscles may be stimulated by massage, heat, and electric current.   32._____
33. Striated muscles are involuntary.   33._____
34. Muscles are always connected directly to bones.   34._____
35. The muscular system relies upon the skeletal and nervous systems for its activities.   35._____
36. Contractility means able to be stretched or extended.   36._____
37. Muscles clothe and support the framework of the body.   37._____
38. The epicranius includes both the occipitalis and frontalis muscles.   38._____
39. The frontalis causes the forehead to wrinkle.   39._____
40. The occipitalis draws the scalp backward.   40._____
41. The levator palpebrae is the muscle that dilates the nostrils.   41._____
42. The orbicularis oculi is the muscle that surrounds the mouth.   42._____
43. The orbicularis oris is the muscle that surrounds the eye.   43._____
44. The trapezius muscle is a muscle of the face.   44._____
45. The temporalis is a muscle of mastication.   45._____
46. The masseter is a muscle that raises the lower jaw against the upper jaw.   46._____
47. The risorius is a muscle that retracts the angle of the mouth.   47._____
48. The sterno-cleido-mastoid muscle depresses and rotates the head.   48._____
49. The platysma is the large muscle in the back of the neck.   49._____
50. The trapezius is the muscle that raises the lower jaw.   50._____
51. The corrugator causes vertical wrinkles at the root of the nose.   51._____
52. The arrector pili is one of the largest muscles of the face.   52._____
53. The epicranius controls the movements of the scalp and wrinkles the forehead.   53._____

54. Muscles of the mouth are supplied by the facial nerve.   54._____

55. The deltoid muscle is a muscle of the lower back.   55._____

KEY (CORRECT ANSWERS)

1. T	11. T	21. T	31. T	41. F	51. T
2. T	12. T	22. F	32. T	42. F	52. F
3. F	13. F	23. T	33. F	43. F	53. T
4. F	14. F	24. F	34. F	44. F	54. T
5. F	15. T	25. T	35. T	45. T	55. F
6. T	16. F	26. T	36. F	46. T	
7. F	17. F	27. T	37. T	47. T	
8. T	18. T	28. F	38. T	48. T	
9. T	19. F	29. T	39. T	49. F	
10. T	20. F	30. F	40. T	50. F	

TEST 3

DIRECTIONS: Fill in the blanks with the MOST appropriate word from the set of words at the beginning of each section. Each answer may be used only once.

Questions 1-10.

tissues   circulatory   skeletal   growth
tendons   reproduction   muscular   nervous
cells   respiratory   organs   glandular

1. Fibrous tissues which connect muscles with bones are called _____.   1.____
2. The cytoplasm of the cell is essential for _____ and the nucleus is essential for _____.   2.____
3. Tissues are combinations of similar _____.   3.____
4. Organs are groups of two or more _____.   4.____
5. Systems are groups of _____.   5.____
6. The physical foundation of the body is the _____ system.   6.____
7. Contraction and movement are characteristic of _____ tissue.   7.____
8. The _____ system coordinates bodily functions.   8.____
9. The _____ system carries food to tissues and waste products from them.   9.____
10. The _____ system purifies the blood by the removal of carbon dioxide gas and the intake of oxygen gas.   10.____

Questions 11-20.

ligaments   flat   gristle   cancellous
mineral   dense   strength   immovable
sphenoid   shape   lacrimal   periosteum
cartilage   muscle   marrow   endosteum

11. Bone is composed of two-thirds _____ matter.   11.____
12. Bones are covered by a thin membrane known as _____.   12.____
13. The functions of the bones are to give _____ and _____ to the body.   13.____
14. The ends of bones are covered with _____.   14.____
15. The skull has _____ shaped bones and _____ joints.   15.____
16. The bone which joins all the bones of the cranium is the _____.   16.____
17. The _____ bones are the smallest and most fragile bones of the face.   17.____
18. Another name for cartilage is _____.   18.____

19. _____ are strong flexible or fibrous tissue that help to hold the bones together at the joints. 19.___

20. There are two types of bone tissue, namely _____ and _____. 20.___

Questions 21-28.

tendons	fascia	trapezius	aponeurosis
500	will	gristle	voluntary
fixed	myology	movable	mandible

21. The origin of a muscle refers to the more _____ attachment; whereas the insertion of a muscle applies to the more _____ attachment. 21.___

22. There are about _____ muscles in the body. 22.___

23. Muscles are joined to bones by means of glistening cords called _____. 23.___

24. A flat expanded tendon which serves to connect one muscle with another is called an _____. 24.___

25. A _____ is a membrane covering and separating layers of muscles. 25.___

26. The muscle which draws the head backward and sideways is the _____. 26.___

27. Voluntary muscles are put into action by the _____. 27.___

28. _____ is the study of the muscles. 28.___

Questions 29-38.

brain	cerebrospinal	digestion	blood
occipital	involuntary	maxillary	glands
muscles	sympathetic	trochlear	nerve
olfactory	mandibular	voluntary	accessory

29. Every muscle has its own _____ and _____ supply. 29.___

30. Sensory nerves carry impulses from the sense organs to the _____. 30.___

31. Motor nerves carry impulses from the brain to the _____. 31.___

32. The cerebrospinal nervous system controls the movements of _____ muscles. 32.___

33. The sympathetic nervous system controls the movements of _____ muscles. 33.___

34. The _____ nerve controls the movement of the superior oblique muscle of the eye. 34.___

35. The posterior auricular nerve supplies the _____ muscle. 35.___

36. The three main branches of the trigeminal nerve are the _____, _____, and _____. 36.___

3 (#3)

37. The _____ system is under the control of the conscious will.   37._____

38. The _____ system controls the functions of circulation, digestion, and secretion of _____.   38._____

Questions 39-50.

superior vena cava	filtration	chest	oxygen
pulmonary veins	arteries	lungs	atrium
pulmonary arteries	ventricle	aorta	inferior
capillaries	bacteria	auricle	liquid

39. The main artery of the body is the _____.   39._____

40. _____ connect the smaller arteries with the veins.   40._____

41. The pulmonary circulation is the blood traveling to and from the heart and _____.   41._____

42. The red blood corpuscles carry _____ to the cells.   42._____

43. White blood cells destroy and devour harmful _____.   43._____

44. Plasma is the _____ portion of the blood.   44._____

45. Lymph is derived from the plasma of the blood by _____.   45._____

46. The upper chamber of the heart is called _____ or _____ and the lower chamber is known as a _____.   46._____

47. Vessels which carry blood from the extremities to the heart are called _____.   47._____

48. Vessels which carry blood from the heart to the lungs are called _____.   48._____

49. Vessels which carry blood from the lungs to the heart are called _____.   49._____

50. Vessels which carry blood from the heart to all parts of the body are called _____.   50._____

KEY (CORRECT ANSWERS)

1. tendons
2. growth, reproduction
3. cells
4. tissues
5. organs

6. skeletal
7. muscular
8. nervous
9. circulatory
10. respiratory

11. mineral
12. periosteum
13. strength, shape
14. cartilage
15. flat, immovable

16. sphenoid
17. lacrimal
18. gristle
19. ligaments
20. dense, cancellous

21. fixed, movable
22. 500
23. tendons
24. aponeurosis
25. fascia

26. trapezius
27. will
28. myology
29. nerve, blood
30. brain

31. muscles
32. voluntary
33. involuntary
34. trochlear
35. occipital

36. ophthalmic, maxillary, mandibular
37. cerebrospinal
38. sympathetic, glands
39. aorta
40. capillaries

41. lungs
42. oxygen
43. bacteria
44. liquid
45. filtration

46. atrium, auricle, ventricle
47. inferior, superior
48. pulmonary arteries
49. pulmonary veins
50. arteries

TEST 4

DIRECTIONS: In each set of questions, match the descriptions in Column II with the appropriate item in Column I. *PRINT THE LETTER OF THE CORRECT ANSWER IN THE SPACE AT THE RIGHT.*

COLUMN I	COLUMN II	

Questions 1-5. Joints.

1. Condyloid	A. Spine	1.____
2. Hinge	B. Neck	2.____
3. Gliding	C. Wrist	3.____
4. Ball and socket	D. Hips	4.____
5. Pivot	E. Elbows	5.____

Questions 6-11. Cranial Bones.

6. Frontal	A. Between the orbits	6.____
7. Sphenoid	B. Ear region	7.____
8. Occipital	C. Crown of head	8.____
9. Ethmoid	D. Forehead	9.____
10. Temporal	E. Base of skull	10.____
11. Parietal	F. Base or brain and back of orbit	11.____

Questions 12-16. Facial Bones.

12. Malar	A. Cheek	12.____
13. Mandible	B. Septum of nose	13.____
14. Nasal	C. Upper jaw	14.____
15. Maxillae	D. Bridge of nose	15.____
16. Vomer	E. Lower jaw	16.____

COLUMN I

COLUMN II

Questions 17-23. Terms.

17.	Anterior	A.	On the side	17.	___
18.	Superior	B.	Situated lower	18.	___
19.	Posterior	C.	Situated higher	19.	___
20.	Inferior	D.	In front of	20.	___
21.	Levator	E.	In back of	21.	___
22.	Lateral	F.	That which enlarges	22.	___
23.	Dilator	G.	That which lifts	23.	___

Questions 24-29. Location of Muscles.

24.	Orbicularis oris	A.	Eyeball	24.	___
25.	Epicranius	B.	Ear	25.	___
26.	Rectus superior	C.	Neck	26.	___
27.	Procerus	D.	Scalp	27.	___
28.	Superior auricular	E.	Mouth	28.	___
29.	Platysma	F.	Nose	29.	___

Questions 30-37. Function of Muscles.

30.	Orbicularis oculi	A.	Opens eye	30.	___
31.	Orbicularis oris	B.	Rotates head	31.	___
32.	Levator palpebrae	C.	Rotates eyeball	32.	___
33.	Rectus muscle	D.	Wrinkles forehead	33.	___
34.	Depressor septi	E.	Contracts cheeks	34.	___
35.	Buccinator	F.	Opens and closes mouth	35.	___
36.	Sterno-cleido-mastoideus	G.	Closes eye	36.	___
37.	Epicranius	H.	Contracts nostrils	37.	___

COLUMN I

Questions 38-44. Function of Nerves.

38.	Olfactory	
39.	Trigeminal	
40.	Glossopharyngeal	
41.	Accessory	
42.	Optic	
43.	Oculomotor	
44.	Auditory	

Questions 45-52. Distribution of Nerves.

45. Infraorbital
46. Mental
47. Supraorbital
48. Palpebral
49. Lingual
50. Nasociliary
51. Auriculo-temporal
52. Ciliary

Questions 53-59. Terms.

53. Atrium
54. Fibrinogen
55. Hemoglobin
56. Lymphatics
57. Ventricle
58. Veins
59. Pericardium

COLUMN II

A. Sensory nerve of sight   38.____
B. Sensory-motor nerve of face and muscles of mastication   39.____
C. Sensory nerve of hearing   40.____
D. Controls movement of eyes   41.____
E. Sensory nerve of smell   42.____
F. Sensory-motor nerve of taste 43.____
G. Controls movement of trapezius muscle   44.____

A. Upper eyelid and forehead   45.____
B. Cornea and iris   46.____
C. Lower lip and chin   47.____
D. Nose   48.____
E. Nose and upper lip   49.____
F. Lower eyelids   50.____
G. Side of scalp   51.____
H. Tongue   52.____

A. A membrane enclosing the heart   53.____
B. Vessels which convey lymph   54.____
C. Upper cavity of the heart   55.____
D. Blood vessels containing valves 56.____
E. Coloring matter of red blood corpuscles   57.____
                                    58.____
F. A substance essential for coagulation of blood   59.____
G. Lower cavity of the heart

COLUMN I	COLUMN II	
Questions 60-65. Distribution of Blood Vessels.		
60. Orbital	A. Back of ears and scalp	60.___
61. Septal	B. Deeper portion of face	61.___
62. Posterior auricular	C. Neck and back part of scalp	62.___
63. Superior labial	D. Nostrils	63.___
64. Occipital	E. Eye cavity	64.___
65. Internal maxillary	F. Upper lip	65.___

KEY (CORRECT ANSWERS)

1.	C	16.	B	31.	F	46.	C	61.	D
2.	E	17.	D	32.	A	47.	A	62.	A
3.	A	18.	C	33.	C	48.	F	63.	F
4.	D	19.	E	34.	H	49.	H	64.	C
5.	B	20.	B	35.	E	50.	D	65.	B
6.	D	21.	G	36.	B	51.	G		
7.	F	22.	A	37.	D	52.	B		
8.	E	23.	F	38.	E	53.	C		
9.	A	24.	E	39.	B	54.	F		
10.	B	25.	D	40.	F	55.	E		
11.	C	26.	A	41.	G	56.	B		
12.	A	27.	F	42.	A	57.	G		
13.	E	28.	B	43.	D	58.	D		
14.	D	29.	C	44.	C	59.	A		
15.	C	30.	G	45.	E	60.	E		

EXAMINATION SECTION
TEST 1

DIRECTIONS: Each question or incomplete statement is followed by several suggested answers or completions. Select the one that BEST answers the question or completes the statement. *PRINT THE LETTER OF THE CORRECT ANSWER IN THE SPACE AT THE RIGHT.*

1. The basic functional unit of life is called a   1._____

    A. nerve
    B. cell
    C. molecule
    D. tendon

2. The study of the organization of tissues is called   2._____

    A. cytology
    B. embryology
    C. histology
    D. anatomy

3. Which of the following organelles plays a critical role in energy production in a eukaryotic cell?   3._____

    A. mitochondria
    B. Golgi apparatus
    C. nucleus
    D. ribosome

4. Which of the following is NOT a structure outside the cell wall?   4._____

    A. capsule
    B. flagella
    C. fimbriae
    D. endoplasmic reticulum

5. The most conspicuous organelle in a eukaryotic cell is the   5._____

    A. mitochondria
    B. nucleus
    C. Golgi apparatus
    D. ribosome

6. The region of the human body which contains the heart, lung, esophagus, thymus and pleura is the

A. abdomen
B. thorax
C. pelvis
D. neck

6._____

7. The thyroid is part of the _____ system.

A. circulatory
B. respiratory
C. endocrine
D. lymphatic

7._____

8. Which of the following is an autoimmune disorder whereby the body's own immune system reacts with the thyroid tissues in an attempt to destroy it?

A. postpartum thyroiditis
B. Hashimoto's disease
C. hypothyroidism
D. hyperthyroidism

8._____

9. The system of the body that contributes to balance and sense of spatial orientation is the _____ system.

A. vestibular
B. nervous
C. musculoskeletal
D. integumenary

9._____

10. An electrically excitable cell that processes and transmits information by electrical and chemical signaling is called a

A. synapse
B. tendon
C. neuron
D. tissue

10._____

11. How many bones does the hand contain?

A. 14
B. 22
C. 27
D. 31

11._____

12. Contractile tissue of animals derived from the mesodermal layer of embryonic germ cell is

A. tendon
B. muscle
C. bone
D. joint

12._____

13. The body part that forms the supporting structure of a human being is the

A. tendon
B. muscle
C. dermis
D. skeleton

13._____

14. The longest bone in the human body is the

A. patella
B. ulna
C. humerus
D. femur

14._____

15. The part of the body made up by the cervical, thoracic, and lumbar vertebrae is the

A. head
B. spine
C. arm
D. leg

15._____

16. All of the following are facial bones EXCEPT

A. phalanges
B. frontal
C. parietal
D. mandible

16._____

17. The human body is composed of approximately _____ muscles.

A. 125
B. 350
C. 640
D. 710

17._____

18. The science of the mechanical, physical, bioelectrical and biochemical functions of humans in good health, their organs and the cells of which they are composed is

A. cytology
B. anatomy
C. physiology
D. embryology

18._____

19. The organ system used for breathing and composed of the pharynx, larynx, trachea, bronchi, lungs and diaphragm is the _____ system.

A. respiratory
B. digestive
C. lymphatic
D. vestibular

19._____

20. The smallest of the body's blood vessels are the

A. veins
B. arteries
C. capillaries
D. villi

20._____

21. Arteries that carry deoxygenated blood to the heart and towards the lungs, where carbon dioxide is exchanged for oxygen are

A. pulmonary arteries
B. systemic arteries
C. arterioles
D. capillaries

21._____

22. An enclosed cable-like bundle of peripheral axons is called a

A. nucleus
B. vein
C. bone
D. nerve

22._____

23. The scientific generic name for a blood cell is a

A. erythrocyte
B. leukocyte
C. hematocyte
D. thrombocyte

23._____

24. Platelets have a lifetime of about 24._____

A. 24 hours
B. 1 day
C. 10 days
D. 1 month

25. Endocrine glands secrete 25._____

A. sweat
B. hormones
C. oils
D. enzymes

KEY (CORRECT ANSWERS)

1. B	6. B	11. C	16. A	21. A
2. C	7. C	12. B	17. C	22. D
3. A	8. B	13. D	18. C	23. C
4. D	9. A	14. D	19. A	24. C
5. B	10. C	15. B	20. C	25. B

TEST 2

DIRECTIONS: Each question or incomplete statement is followed by several suggested answers or completions. Select the one that BEST answers the question or completes the statement. *PRINT THE LETTER OF THE CORRECT ANSWER IN THE SPACE AT THE RIGHT.*

1. A group of unicellular organisms having characteristics of both plant and animals are

    A. fungi
    B. bacteria
    C. parasites
    D. mites

1._____

2. A small infectious agent that can replicate only inside the cells of living organisms is a

    A. spore
    B. dermophyte
    C. virus
    D. parasite

2._____

3. Bacteria can be found

    A. in the ocean
    B. on land
    C. in soil
    D. everywhere on Earth

3._____

4. There are approximately _____ bacteria on earth.

    A. 500 thousand
    B. 500 million
    C. 500 billion
    D. 5 nonillion

4._____

5. All of the following are diseases caused by pathogenic bacteria EXCEPT

    A. cholera
    B. syphilis
    C. influenza
    D. leprosy

5._____

6. Bacteria are now regarded as

    A. prokaryotes
    B. eukaryotes
    C. plants
    D. animals

6._____

7. The first bacteria to be discovered were   7._____

   A. round
   B. rod-shaped
   C. square
   D. triangular

8. Bacteria lack a(n)   8._____

   A. nucleus
   B. Golgi apparatus
   C. Endoplasmic reticulum
   D. all of the above

9. Rigid protein structures that are used for motility are   9._____

   A. flagella
   B. fimbriae
   C. pili
   D. macrophages

10. What kind of energy do phototrophs use?   10._____

    A. sunlight
    B. organic compounds
    C. inorganic compound
    D. oxygen

11. The first phase of bacterial growth is called the _____ phase.   11._____

    A. log
    B. lag
    C. stationary
    D. repair

12. Blood-sucking insects that transmit disease from one organism to another   12._____
are known as

    A. viruses
    B. bacteriae
    C. vectors
    D. parasites

13. Generally, viruses are _____ bacteria.   13._____

    A. smaller than
    B. larger than
    C. the same size as
    D. more abundant than

14. The process by which a strand of DNA is broken and then joined to the end of a different DNA molecule is called

    A. genetic drift
    B. antigenic shift
    C. genetic recombination
    D. viral evolution

15. The process in which the viral capsid is removed is called

    A. attachment
    B. penetration
    C. uncoating
    D. replication

16. A process that kills the cell by bursting its membrane and cell wall if present is called

    A. lysis
    B. budding
    C. penetration
    D. modification

17. Replication of RNA viruses usually takes place in the

    A. nucleus
    B. cytoplasm
    C. Golgi apparatus
    D. endoplasmic reticulum

18. The _____ virus can cause cancer.

    A. herpes
    B. Epstein-Barr
    C. papilloma
    D. human immunodeficiency

19. All of the following are common human diseases caused by viruses EXCEPT

    A. influenza
    B. chicken pox
    C. cold sores
    D. strep throat

20. A biological term that describes a state of having sufficient biological defenses to avoid infection, disease or other unwanted biological invasion is called

   A. bacteriology
   B. immunity
   C. inoculation
   D. safety

20._____

21. T cells belong to a group of white blood cells called

   A. thrombocytes
   B. lymphocytes
   C. leukocytes
   D. erythrocytes

21._____

22. A substance that contains an antigen and is used to artificially acquire active immunity is known as a

   A. platelet
   B. vaccine
   C. serum
   D. venom

22._____

23. Parasitism is a type of _____ relationship between organisms of different species where one organism, the parasite, benefits at the expense of the other, the host.

   A. moral
   B. monogamous
   C. symbiotic
   D. mellifluous

23._____

24. Parasites that live on the surface of the host are called

   A. ectoparasites
   B. endoparasites
   C. epiparasites
   D. brood parasites

24._____

25. The most important measure for preventing the spread of pathogens is effective

   A. vaccination
   B. protective equipment
   C. hand washing
   D. isolation

25._____

KEY (CORRECT ANSWERS)

1. B	6. A	11. B	16. A	21. B
2. C	7. B	12. C	17. B	22. B
3. D	8. D	13. A	18. C	23. C
4. D	9. A	14. C	19. D	24. A
5. C	10. A	15. C	20. B	25. C

SHAMPOOING & SCALP TREATMENTS

EXAMINATION SECTION
TEST 1

DIRECTIONS: Each question consists of a statement. You are to indicate whether the statement is TRUE (T) or FALSE (F). *PRINT THE LETTER OF THE CORRECT ANSWER IN THE SPACE AT THE RIGHT.*

1. Always follow a shampoo with a cool rinse.   1.____
2. The proper way to comb snarls out of the hair is to start combing from the scalp.   2.____
3. A few drops of carbolic acid in the shampoo mixture is recommended for dry hair.   3.____
4. The shades obtained from a henna shampoo will range from reddish brown to dark brown.   4.____
5. Boiling henna leaves for a few minutes, and then straining, will produce a henna rinse.   5.____
6. Pure castile soap is good for a general shampoo.   6.____
7. A tar shampoo is excellent for dry hair.   7.____
8. Hot oil treatment is excellent for corrective purposes.   8.____
9. Frequent shampoos are necessary for a perspiring scalp.   9.____
10. Hair which has turned bright red after a henna rinse should be rinsed with vinegar.   10.____
11. Always stimulate the scalp before each shampoo.   11.____
12. Sage tea is a bleach.   12.____
13. A vinegar rinse will cause hair to snarl.   13.____
14. An egg shampoo is recommended for overbleached hair.   14.____
15. Yellow streaks in white hair may be caused by acid in the system.   15.____
16. Water that is too hot dries the scalp.   16.____
17. Water is composed of hydrogen and oxygen.   17.____
18. Heated oil is not good for general use on the hair.   18.____
19. A peroxide rinse is used to give the hair a reddish tint.   19.____
20. Henna rinse and henna compound have the same base.   20.____
21. Tar shampoos are advised for light hair only.   21.____
22. Egg shampoos are advised for bleached, dry, and brittle hair.   22.____
23. Bleached hair should be rinsed with very hot water.   23.____

24. A rinse may mean any liquid used to remove soap. 24.____

25. Colored rinses penetrate the hair shaft. 25.____

26. Castile soap is usually made of linseed oil and an alkali. 26.____

27. A thorough cleansing shampoo aids in maintaining the hygiene of hair and scalp. 27.____

28. The frequency of shampoos depends on the season of the year. 28.____

29. Dry hair requires more frequent shampoos than oily hair. 29.____

30. When a shampoo is mixed with hard water, it produces a copious lather. 30.____

31. Hard water contains the soluble salts of calcium and magnesium in solution. 31.____

32. A dry shampoo cleanses the hair by absorbing the dirt and oil. 32.____

33. Coconut oil is a desirable ingredient in shampoos because it helps to form a thick lather. 33.____

34. A gasoline shampoo is dangerous because it is inflammable. 34.____

35. Vinegar and lemon rinses help to neutralize the alkaline soap residue on the hair and scalp. 35.____

KEY (CORRECT ANSWERS)

1.	T	16.	T
2.	F	17.	T
3.	F	18.	F
4.	F	19.	F
5.	T	20.	T
6.	T	21.	F
7.	F	22.	T
8.	T	23.	F
9.	T	24.	T
10.	F	25.	F
11.	T	26.	F
12.	F	27.	T
13.	F	28.	F
14.	T	29.	F
15.	T	30.	F

31. T
32. T
33. T
34. T
35. T

TEST 2

Questions 1-5.

DIRECTIONS: Each question consists of a statement. You are to indicate whether the statement is TRUE (T) or FALSE (F). *PRINT THE LETTER OF THE CORRECT ANSWER IN THE SPACE AT THE RIGHT.*

1. In the treatment for eczema of the scalp, the hair should be combed without scraping or scratching the scalp. 1.____

2. The most hygienic way to stimulate the circulation of the scalp is by scratching it. 2.____

3. In the treatment for alopecia, the high-frequency current is applied with a glass rake electrode but without sparks. 3.____

4. The cosmetologist is most concerned with the treatment of scalp diseases. 4.____

5. A shampoo rarely accompanies a scalp treatment. 5.____

Questions 6-25.

DIRECTIONS: Fill in the blanks with the most appropriate word from the set of words at the beginning of each section. Each answer may be used only once.

Questions 6-15.

supraorbital	shampoo	growth	cleanses
stimulates	rotary	brittle	frontal
manipulations	occipital	full	lustre
underneath	antiseptic	scalp	dry

6. Scalp manipulations increase the _____ and _____ of the hair by way of improved circulation and nutrition. 6.____

7. Although the hair is cleansed by means of a shampoo, it will not prevent the hair from becoming _____ and _____. 7.____

8. The operator should wash her hands in an _____ solution before and after administering scalp treatments. 8.____

9. The same scalp _____ are applied to all scalp treatments. 9.____

10. Massaging the scalp stimulates the flow of blood through the temporal, auricular, _____, _____, and _____ arteries. 10.____

11. To avoid pulling the hair while massaging the scalp, slide the hands _____ the hair. 11.____

12. _____ scalp manipulations activate cellular metabolism and loosen scalp tissues. 12.____

13. Brushing the hair should always be a part of a _____ and most of _____ treatments. 13.____

14. Brushing the hair is beneficial because it _____ the scalp and _____ the hair. 14.____

79

15. The bristles of the brush are held against the scalp and are swept the _____ length of the hair.   15.____

Questions 16-25.

erythema	ultra-violet	sulphur	egg
high-frequency	alopecia	growth	spots
electrode	scraping	sunburn	dry
scratching	sparking	eczema	after

16. Both the _____ current and _____ rays are employed in the treatment for dandruff.   16.____

17. A _____ scalp may be caused by frequent washing of the hair with a strong soap.   17.____

18. An _____ shampoo is used to cleanse a dry and tender scalp.   18.____

19. When hair tonics are used in connection with high-frequency, they must be applied _____ using the current.   19.____

20. A treatment for alopecia is designed to stimulate the _____ of the hair.   20.____

21. In alopecia areata, baldness appears in _____.   21.____

22. _____ ointment is recommended for the treatment of alopecia areata and eczema of the scalp.   22.____

23. Irradiating the scalp with ultra-violet rays for a period of five minutes will produce a first degree _____ or _____.   23.____

24. In the treatment for alopecia, apply the high-frequency current directly to the scalp with a glass rake _____ and without _____.   24.____

25. In dressing the hair after a scalp treatment, avoid _____ or _____ the scalp with the comb.   25.____

Questions 26-30.

DIRECTIONS: In each set of questions, match the items in Column II with the appropriate item in Column I. *PRINT THE LETTER OF THE CORRECT ANSWER IN THE SPACE AT THE RIGHT.*

COLUMN I		COLUMN II	
26. Anoint	A.	Dandruff	26.____
27. Erythema	B.	Hair dressing	27.____
28. Pomade	C.	Expose to natural or artificial sunlight	28.____
29. Irradiate	D.	Application of oil or cream to the skin	29.____
30. Pityriasis	E.	Redness of the skin	30.____

KEY (CORRECT ANSWERS)

1. T
2. F
3. T
4. F
5. F
6. growth, lustre
7. dry, brittle
8. antiseptic
9. manipulations
10. occipital, supraorbital, frontal
11. underneath
12. rotary
13. shampoo, scalp
14. stimulates, cleanses
15. full
16. high-frequency, ultra-violet
17. dry
18. egg
19. after
20. growth
21. spots
22. sulphur
23. erythema, sunburn
24. electrode, sparking
25. scraping, scratching
26. D
27. E
28. B
29. C
30. A

HAIRCUTTING, CURLING & WAVING
EXAMINATION SECTION
TEST 1

DIRECTIONS: Each question consists of a statement. You are to indicate whether the statement is TRUE (T) or FALSE (F). *PRINT THE LETTER OF THE CORRECT ANSWER IN THE SPACE AT THE RIGHT.*

1. Hair should never be thinned close to the scalp. 1.____
2. Effileing and slithering are the same. 2.____
3. A cowlick is caused by a scalp disease. 3.____
4. Thinning is always done with thinning shears. 4.____
5. A razor is never used for tapering and thinning. 5.____
6. Neck dusters are never sterilized. 6.____
7. It is advisable to singe the hair before shampooing. 7.____
8. Hair is always shampooed before cutting. 8.____
9. The treatment for trichoptilosis is clipping or singeing. 9.____
10. Alcohol may be used for sterilizing clippers and shears. 10.____
11. Bangs are best suited to a face with a high forehead. 11.____
12. The hair should be thinned before a marcel wave. 12.____
13. Pointed necklines are suggested for long, slender necks. 13.____
14. The principal difference between a shingle bob and a feather-edge is the height at which the hair is cut. 14.____
15. The thumb is uppermost on the scissors when shingling or feather-edging. 15.____
16. In singeing the hair, the lighted taper is passed over loose hair. 16.____
17. A correct haircut will emphasize the attractive features and minimize the defects. 17.____
18. A number one hair clipper makes the shortest cut. 18.____
19. A good hair comb is made of hard rubber. 19.____
20. Use a fresh neck strip and towel for each customer. 20.____
21. If a mistake is made in marcelling, it can be corrected. 21.____
22. The marcel wave was created by Francois Marcel to imitate naturally wavy hair. 22.____
23. French paper curls are advised for thick, coarse hair. 23.____

24. Round curls give a fluffy effect to fine, thin hair. 24._____
25. Marcel waves should never be brushed. 25._____
26. A hot iron should never be used when marcelling gray hair. 26._____
27. A Francois Marcel and croquignole marcel are given in the same way. 27._____
28. Marcelling cannot be accomplished with kinky hair. 28._____
29. It is not necessary to stretch the hair in order to produce a lasting wave. 29._____
30. It is necessary to use a hot iron on bleached hair. 30._____
31. The temperature of the irons should not be the same for every texture of hair. 31._____
32. Medium warm irons are employed for croquignole marcel waving. 32._____
33. Start a croquignole marcel wave at the back of the head. 33._____
34. In marcelling, the hair should be picked up with a comb, not with an iron. 34._____
35. Brushing and combing injure marcel waves. 35._____
36. To become skillful in finger waving, the operator should rely on mechanical aids. 36._____
37. Always start a finger wave at the back of the head. 37._____
38. Finger waving is easier to accomplish if the proper waving lotion is used. 38._____
39. The hair should be thoroughly combed before finger waving. 39._____
40. After the finger wave is formed, it is not necessary to reset waves into a soft coiffure. 40._____

KEY (CORRECT ANSWERS)

1.	T	11.	F	21.	T	31.	T
2.	T	12.	T	22.	T	32.	T
3.	F	13.	F	23.	F	33.	F
4.	F	14.	T	24.	T	34.	T
5.	F	15.	F	25.	F	35.	F
6.	F	16.	F	26.	T	36.	F
7.	T	17.	T	27.	F	37.	F
8.	F	18.	F	28.	F	38.	T
9.	T	19.	T	29.	F	39.	T
10.	T	20.	T	30.	F	40.	F

TEST 2

DIRECTIONS: Each question consists of a statement. You are to indicate whether the statement is TRUE (T) or FALSE (F). *PRINT THE LETTER OF THE CORRECT ANSWER IN THE SPACE AT THE RIGHT.*

1. In giving a machineless permanent wave, the steaming time given to all textures of hair is the same, but the solution varies. 1.____

2. Fine hair has more elasticity than coarse hair. 2.____

3. Dyed hair should be steamed longer than normal hair. 3.____

4. A full twist will give a marcel effect while a flat wrap will give a round curl effect on a spiral wrap permanent. 4.____

5. The steaming time on fine and coarse hair is the same, providing the wrap is different. 5.____

6. All systems of heat permanents are dependent upon moisture, alkali, contraction, and expansion of the hair. 6.____

7. Average healthy hair can be stretched about twenty percent of its own length. 7.____

8. The hydroscopic quality of hair means its ability to absorb liquids. 8.____

9. When hair becomes too kinky from a permanent wave, hot oil treatments will help. 9.____

10. Less time is given to steaming fine hair than coarse hair. 10.____

11. A permanent wave can be given successfully over a head of bleached hair. 11.____

12. The hair ends are wrapped closer to the nape of the neck in a croquignole winding. 12.____

13. Moisture absorbed by the hair in permanent waving causes the hair to expand. 13.____

14. Improper wrapping causes hair to break. 14.____

15. Always put on sachets while dripping wet. 15.____

16. A spiral flat wrap on long hair is never overlapped. 16.____

17. You can successfully permanent wave over henna. 17.____

18. If a dye and a permanent wave are to be given, the dye should be given first. 18.____

19. A loose wave is always obtained by less steaming. 19.____

20. Hair nearest the head is hardest to soften with permanent waving solution. 20.____

21. Borax solution will always cause white or gray hair to turn yellow. 21.____

22. A vinegar rinse sometimes strengthens a permanent wave. 22.____

23. Blonde hair sometimes changes color in permanent waving. 23.____

24. Elasticity of hair is weakened by bleaching. 24.____

25. Oversteamed hair can be restored to its original texture. 25.____

26. All bleached hair can be given a successful permanent wave. 26.____

27. The width of the wave depends upon the amount of hair used in each strand. 27.____

28. A successful permanent wave can be given over a hair restorer. 28.____

29. It is better to oversteam than to understeam the hair. 29.____

30. It is always advisable to make a test curl. 30.____

31. Hair of a porous nature is the most difficult to wave. 31.____

32. A vinegar rinse will help to remove snarls occasioned by oversteamed or kinky hair. 32.____

33. In a croquignole permanent wave, the protectors are attached to the head before the hair is wound. 33.____

34. There is no difference between a wet and dry winding since both are treated with pads. 34.____

35. A spiral permanent wave is usually wound from the hair ends to the scalp. 35.____

KEY (CORRECT ANSWERS)

1.	T	11.	T	21.	T	31.	F
2.	F	12.	F	22.	F	32.	T
3.	F	13.	T	23.	T	33.	T
4.	F	14.	T	24.	T	34.	F
5.	F	15.	F	25.	F	35.	F
6.	T	16.	F	26.	F		
7.	T	17.	T	27.	T		
8.	T	18.	F	28.	F		
9.	T	19.	T	29.	F		
10.	F	20.	T	30.	T		

TEST 3

DIRECTIONS: Fill in the blanks with the MOST appropriate word from the set of words at the beginning of each section. Each answer may be used only once.

Questions 1-12.

dryer	condition	guarantee	floor
record	texture	hair	oil
patron	thinning	cords	clips
warm	protectors	dry	cold
prior	preliminary	scalp	brittle
reconditioning	excessively	test	tight

1. Always examine the patron's _____ and _____ and take _____ curls before a wave. 1.____

2. Avoid electric shock by keeping the hands, electrical _____ and _____ under machine in a _____ condition. 2.____

3. Keep a _____ of every permanent wave given. 3.____

4. Never leave a _____ unattended while giving a permanent wave. 4.____

5. The strength of the softener and length of steaming time must be adjusted to the _____ and _____ of the patron's hair. 5.____

6. Do not attempt to wave dry, brittle, bleached or dyed hair without _____ the hair with _____ treatments. 6.____

7. Shape the hair _____ to waving. Heavy hair needs _____. 7.____

8. Prevent scalp and pull burn bruises by using felts, _____, and _____. 8.____

9. Cool hair under _____ before unwinding it. 9.____

10. Give a _____ shampoo to dyed or bleached hair only when it is _____ oily. 10.____

11. Rinse tight curls with _____ water and loose curls with _____ water. 11.____

12. Do not _____ the success of a permanent wave. 12.____

Questions 13-25.

slightly	each	hot oil	very fine
curlers	tight	softener	two inches
spiral	wound	rod	flat
croquignole	brittle	heaters	felts
before	waving	open heater	beneficial
varies	softener	marcel wave	closed heater
spiral	croquignole	long	one inch

2 (#3)

13. Scalp and _____ treatments are _____ in keeping the hair soft and silky. 13._____

14. Consult manufacturers' instructions for correct use of machine, _____ or _____. 14._____

15. In a wet spiral wind, the hair is wetted with _____ first, then wound around the _____. 15._____

16. In a dry spiral wind, the hair is _____ first. 16._____

17. A wet wind requires a _____ for steaming while a dry wind requires an _____ for steaming. 17._____

18. Wet wind is preferred for _____ hair. 18._____

19. A flat type wind produces a _____ effect. 19._____

20. For croquignole winding, section the hair about _____ wide and _____ long. 20._____

21. In croquignole winding, use a wet wrap by moistening hair with _____ lotion and winding the hair absolutely _____ around rod. 21._____

22. In croquignole waving, the sachets are wetted _____ and then wrapped around _____. 22._____

23. In combination permanent waving, the top hair is wound in a _____ fashion. The hair at the sides and back of the head is given a _____ wind. 23._____

24. In combination permanent waving, both _____ and _____ test curls are given _____ waving the entire head. 24._____

25. In combination permanent waving, steaming time _____ on _____ part of the head. 25._____

Questions 26-35.

fine	bleached	dyes	tinted
over-steaming	brittle	saturated	changed
metallic	neutralized	waving	texture
coarse	not	condition	stretching

26. Recondition dry, _____ hair before giving a cold wave. 26._____

27. The hair must be thoroughly _____ with the _____ solution. 27._____

28. In cold waving, wind hair smoothly without _____. 28._____

29. In cold waving, in order to set the hair it must be thoroughly _____. 29._____

30. Examine the hair carefully to judge its _____ and _____. 30._____

31. In heat waving, structure of the hair is _____ while in cold waving the structure and texture of the hair is _____ changed. 31._____

32. Cold waves can be applied to hair of any texture or to hair previously _____, _____ or waved. 32._____

33. As in heat waving, cold waves cannot be given to hair that has been treated with metallic _____ or rinses. 33._____

34. In heat waving, _____ hair is easiest to wave, while in cold waving _____ hair is easiest to wave. 34._____

35. Stretching in cold waving is equivalent to _____ in heat waving. 35._____

Questions 36-40.

thick	thin	inside	light
10	15	heavy	bottom
net	outside	cellophane wrap	down

36. Start the finger wave on the _____ or _____ side of the hair. 36._____

37. Combs and brushes should be sterilized in _____ % formalin solution. 37._____

38. In a pin curl, the hair ends are on the _____ of the curl. 38._____

39. In a sculpture curl, the hair ends are on the _____ of the curl. 39._____

40. While the hair is being dried, it should be kept in place with a _____ . 40._____

DIRECTIONS: In the following set of questions, match the descriptions in Column II with the appropriate item in Column I. *PRINT THE LETTER OF THE CORRECT ANSWER IN THE SPACE AT THE RIGHT.*

COLUMN I

41. Wave curl
42. Sculpture curl
43. Brush curl
44. Pin curl
45. Hair line curl

COLUMN II

A. Hair is wound so that hair ends are on inside of curl.
B. Hair is wound so that hair ends are on outside of curl.
C. Hair ends are wound in concentric circles toward the scalp.
D. Hair is wound to form an overlapping curl.
E. Each succeeding circle is placed inside of the previous circle.

41._____
42._____
43._____
44._____
45._____

KEY (CORRECT ANSWERS)

1. scalp, hair, test
2. cords, floor, dry
3. record
4. patron
5. texture, condition

6. reconditioning, oil
7. prior, thinning
8. protectors, clips
9. dryer
10. preliminary, excessively

11. warm, cold
12. guarantee
13. hot oil, beneficial
14. softener, heaters
15. softener, rod

16. wound
17. closed heater, open heater
18. very fine
19. marcel wave
20. one inch, two inches

21. waving, flat
22. slightly, curlers
23. spiral, croquignole
24. spiral, croquignole, before
25. varies, each

26. brittle
27. saturated, waving
28. stretching
29. neutralized
30. texture, condition

31. changed, not
32. bleached, tinted
33. dyes
34. fine, coarse
35. over-steaming

36. thick, heavy
37. 10
38. outside
39. inside
40. net

41. E
42. A
43. D
44. B
45. C

FACIALS AND MANICURING

EXAMINATION SECTION
TEST 1

DIRECTIONS: Each question consists of a statement. You are to indicate whether the statement is TRUE (T) or FALSE (F). *PRINT THE LETTER OF THE CORRECT ANSWER IN THE SPACE AT THE RIGHT.*

1. Correct massage is given by stretching the skin in an upward and downward direction. 1._____
2. The loss of elasticity of the muscles will cause wrinkles. 2._____
3. Tapotement is the slapping movement. 3._____
4. Large pores in the skin are caused by the use of good astringents. 4._____
5. Skin bleaching lubricates the skin. 5._____
6. Heat causes the skin to contract. 6._____
7. Facials may be given once a week if necessary. 7._____
8. Vanishing creams are non-absorbent and serve as a powder base. 8._____
9. Fine skin requires less cleansing treatments than coarse skin. 9._____
10. Astringent lotion lubricates the underlying tissues. 10._____
11. Makeup of all kinds should correspond to the natural coloring of the individual. 11._____
12. Cleansing creams are absorbed by the skin. 12._____
13. Tissue cream is used to nourish the skin. 13._____
14. A double chin is due to a lack of adipose tissue. 14._____
15. All eyebrows should be arched the same way. 15._____
16. Petrissage is a kneading movement. 16._____
17. A clay pack tends to expand the skin tissue. 17._____
18. A sudden loss of weight may be responsible for wrinkles. 18._____
19. Lanolin is a beneficial ingredient in tissue creams. 19._____
20. The eyes should be covered with pads when exposing the face to therapeutic lights. 20._____
21. The matrix is the reproductive organ of the nail. 21._____
22. The nail receives its nourishment from the matrix during growth. 22._____
23. The nail bed is composed of the same layers as the corium of the skin. 23._____

24. The shape of the nail is determined by the shape of the finger. 24.___
25. The nail should be filed from the center to the corners. 25.___
26. Hangnails are a splitting of the epidermis at the side of the finger. 26.___
27. Liquid polish is injurious to the nail. 27.___
28. Onychophagy should be treated as a disease. 28.___
29. Nails filed long and given oil manicures will aid in keeping them from splitting. 29.___
30. Onychia is inflammation of the nail matrix. 30.___
31. If a nail is torn, cut or injured, a new one will always grow. 31.___
32. A styptic pencil is used to stop bleeding from a minor cut or abrasion. 32.___
33. The nails contain numerous cells joined together to form epithelial tissue. 33.___
34. The matrix extends beneath the nail root. 34.___
35. Onychosis is ringworm of the nail. 35.___
36. Leuconychia is white spots in the nail. 36.___
37. A hand and arm massage can be given both for thin and fat hands. 37.___
38. Paronychia is a non-infectious disease of the nails. 38.___
39. Chapped hands are caused by frequent washing and exposure to the cold. 39.___
40. The cuticle of the nail is the same as the outside of the hair. 40.___
41. The nail is very thick in the region of the root. 41.___
42. Hot oil manicures are beneficial for ridged and brittle nails. 42.___
43. Nail infections are caused by sterilized instruments. 43.___
44. A sharp instrument should never be used to push back the cuticle. 44.___
45. Digital nerves are not branches of the radial and ulnar nerves. 45.___
46. Buffing is always a part of the manicure when a liquid polish is not to be used. 46.___
47. Abrasions are less likely to result with an orangewood stick than with a metal cleaner. 47.___
48. The color of a healthy nail is white. 48.___
49. Corns should be removed when giving a pedicure. 49.___
50. Alcohol is a good remedy for perspiring hands. 50.___

KEY (CORRECT ANSWERS)

1. F	11. T	21. T	31. F	41. F
2. T	12. F	22. T	32. F	42. T
3. T	13. T	23. T	33. F	43. F
4. F	14. F	24. T	34. T	44. T
5. F	15. F	25. F	35. F	45. F
6. F	16. T	26. T	36. T	46. T
7. T	17. F	27. F	37. T	47. T
8. T	18. T	28. F	38. F	48. F
9. F	19. T	29. T	39. T	49. F
10. F	20. T	30. T	40. F	50. T

TEST 2

Questions 1-4.

DIRECTIONS: Each question consists of a statement. You are to indicate whether the statement is TRUE (T) or FALSE (F). *PRINT THE LETTER OF THE CORRECT ANSWER IN THE SPACE AT THE RIGHT.*

1. Hydrogen peroxide solution is used as a germicide in manicuring.   1._____

2. The nail blade has a vascular supply while the matrix has none.   2._____

3. Muscle toning treatments are recommended for oily skin.   3._____

4. Massage helps to eliminate the waste products of metabolism.   4._____

Questions 5-14.

DIRECTIONS: Fill in the blanks with the MOST appropriate word from the set of words at the beginning of each section. Each answer may be used only once.

file	sterilized	convex	free edge
new	arranged	old	centers
dry	infections	long	nail bed
short	sanitary	brittle	blemishes

5. Manicuring beautifies the nails and keeps them in a _____ condition.   5._____

6. An efficient manicurist keeps her instruments properly _____ and conveniently _____ so that they are readily accessible.   6._____

7. As applied to the shape of nails, concave is the opposite of _____.   7._____

8. Before giving a manicure, the operator should examine the hands for _____ and _____.   8._____

9. If the shape of the nail conforms to the type of finger, then a long, oval-shaped nail should be selected for a _____ stumpy finger.   9._____

10. A manicure starts with the removal of _____ nail polish and ends with the application of a _____ film of nail polish.   10._____

11. Nails are filed from either corner to their _____.   11._____

12. Nail whitening is applied under the _____ of the nail.   12._____

13. The emery board is used in the same manner as the nail _____.   13._____

14. An oil manicure is beneficial for ridged and _____ nails and _____ cuticles.   14._____

Questions 15-35.

DIRECTIONS: In each set of questions, match the items in Column I with the appropriate item in Column I. *PRINT THE LETTER OF THE CORRECT ANSWER IN THE SPACE AT THE RIGHT.*

COLUMN I   COLUMN II

Questions 15-19.

15. Leuconychia   A. Inflammation of the nail matrix with pus formation   15.____
16. Atrophy   16.____
17. Onychia   B. Swelling of the nails   17.____
18. Onychoptosis   C. White spots on the nails   18.____
19. Onychophyma   D. Periodical shedding of the nails   19.____
                         E. Wasting away of the nail

Questions 20-24.

20. Nail body   A. Base of nail imbedded underneath the skin   20.____
21. Nail bed   21.____
22. Nail root   B. Part of nail bed extending beneath nail root   22.____
23. Matrix   C. Overlapping skin around the nail   23.____
24. Cuticle   D. Skin on which nail body rests   24.____
                         E. Nail extending from root to fingertips

Questions 25-30.

25. Humerus   A. Large bone of the forearm   25.____
26. Carpus   B. Small bone of the forearm   26.____
27. Radial blood vessel C. Bones of the wrist   27.____
28. Radius   D. Bone of the upper arm   28.____
29. Phalanges   E. Supplies outer side of arm and back of hand   29.____
30. Ulna   30.____
                         F. Bones of fingers and toes

Questions 31-35.

COLUMN I	COLUMN II	
31. Vibroid	A. Kneading movement	31. ____
32. Friction	B. Tapping movement	32. ____
33. Petrissage	C. Vibratory movement	33. ____
34. Effleurage	D. Deep rubbing movement	34. ____
35. Tapotement	E. Stroking movement	35. ____

KEY (CORRECT ANSWERS)

1. F	11. centers	21. D	31. C
2. F	12. free edge	22. A	32. D
3. F	13. file	23. B	33. A
4. T	14. brittle, dry	24. C	34. E
5. sanitary	15. C	25. D	35. B
6. sterilized, arranged	16. E	26. C	
7. convex	17. A	27. E	
8. blemishes, infections	18. D	28. B	
9. short	19. B	29. F	
10. old, new	20. E	30. A	

ELECTRICITY & LIGHT THERAPY
EXAMINATION SECTION
TEST 1

DIRECTIONS: Each question consists of a statement. You are to indicate whether the statement is TRUE (T) or FALSE (F). *PRINT THE LETTER OF THE CORRECT ANSWER IN THE SPACE AT THE RIGHT.*

1. An alternating current flows first in one direction and then in the opposite direction. 1.____
2. High frequency treatments may be given after an alcohol tonic has been applied. 2.____
3. The colors of the visible spectrum range from deep red through orange, yellow, green, blue, indigo, and violet. 3.____
4. Infra-red rays are purely heat rays. 4.____
5. Ultra-violet rays are chemical rays. 5.____
6. Electricity may be transmitted to the patron through the use of the vibrator. 6.____
7. A rectifier is an apparatus for changing or converting an alternating current into a direct current. 7.____
8. High frequency treatments may not be given after an application of oil. 8.____
9. Copper is never used as a conductor. 9.____
10. Polarity refers to the action of the current entering and leaving the machine. 10.____
11. It is not necessary to test for polarity. 11.____
12. High frequency is an oscillating current, is stimulating, and germicidal. 12.____
13. A closed circuit is one in which a current is continually flowing. 13.____
14. The negative pole of galvanism is alkaline in reaction. 14.____
15. It is unnecessary to sterilize electrodes used with high frequency. 15.____
16. An insulator conveys an electrical current. 16.____
17. The heat element in sunlight is called infra-red. 17.____
18. An ohm is a unit of current resistance. 18.____
19. The infra-red rays have a chemical effect. 19.____
20. Ultra-violet rays may be used by the beautician in giving facial and scalp treatments. 20.____
21. Any substance which carries electricity freely is called a conductor. 21.____
22. Insulation is not always necessary. 22.____

23. A Faradic current is applied through the scalp.   23.____
24. An ampere is a unit of electrical pressure.   24.____
25. A rheostat regulates the strength of a current.   25.____

KEY (CORRECT ANSWERS)

1.	T	11.	F
2.	F	12.	T
3.	T	13.	T
4.	T	14.	T
5.	T	15.	F
6.	F	16.	F
7.	T	17.	T
8.	F	18.	T
9.	F	19.	F
10.	T	20.	T

21. T
22. F
23. F
24. F
25. T

TEST 2

DIRECTIONS: Fill in the blanks with the MOST appropriate word from the set of words at the beginning of each section. Each answer may be used only once.

Questions 1-10.
acids	thermal	conductor	non-conductor
fuse	kilowatt	chemical	milliamperemeter
light	current	complete	electrons
heat	conductors	closed	resistance

1. Electricity in motion can produce magnetic, _____ or_____ effects.   1.____

2. Watery solutions of acids and salts are good _____ of electricity.   2.____

3. The inside of an electric wire acts as a _____ and the outside functions as a _____.   3.____

4. Electricity is a source of _____ and _____.   4.____

5. To operate an electrical appliance, the circuit should be _____ and _____.   5.____

6. A short circuit can be corrected by inserting a new _____.   6.____

7. An electric current flows through a conductor when the pressure is sufficiently great to overcome the _____ of the wire.   7.____

8. The _____ measures the rate of flow of an electric current.   8.____

9. The _____ unit is used to calculate the cost of consuming electrical power in the beauty shop.   9.____

10. _____ refers to the flow of electricity through a conductor.   10.____

Questions 11-19.
rheostat	direct	stimulation	negative
acid	alkaline	alternating	vibration
faradic	galvanic	irritation	stimulating

11. The _____ current is applied through the fingertips.   11.____

12. The operator should test for polarity before applying the _____ current to the body.   12.____

13. The anode of the galvanic current has an _____ reaction, while the cathode has an _____ reaction.   13.____

14. Galvanism is operated on a _____ current, while faradism is operated on _____.   14.____

15. The physiological effects of the sinusoidal current are great _____ with slight _____.   15.____

16. The high-frequency current has a high rate of _____.   16.____

17. The Tesla current produces a _____ effect if the electrode is lifted slightly from the parts being treated.   17.____

18. The _____ pole of the galvanic current is attached to the electrolytic cup.   18.____

19. A _____ regulates current through variable resistances. 19._____

Questions 20-30.
first	frequency	12	glare
blue	ultra-violet	length	red
skin	dermal	infra-red	scalp
heat	spectrum	therapy	30

20. Light therapy is employed in the treatment of _____ and _____ diseases and to keep the body in a healthy condition. 20._____

21. The _____ rays are the shortest and the least penetrating rays of the spectrum. 21._____

22. The _____ rays are the longest and the most penetrating rays of the spectrum. 22._____

23. Different light rays vary in their _____ and _____. 23._____

24. The _____ dermal light is deficient in heat rays. 24._____

25. The _____ light has strong heat rays. 25._____

26. The eyes should be protected from the _____ and _____ of light. 26._____

27. The infra-red lamp is operated at an average distance of _____ inches from the skin. 27._____

28. The ultra-violet lamp should be placed at a distance of _____ inches from the skin. 28._____

29. For cosmetic purposes, a _____ degree sunburn is the safest. 29._____

30. The treatment of a disease or disorder is a type of _____. 30._____

KEY (CORRECT ANSWERS)

1. chemical, thermal
2. conductors
3. conductor, non-conductor
4. light, heat
5. complete, closed

6. fuse
7. resistance
8. milliamperemeter
9. kilowatt
10. current

11. faradic
12. galvanic
13. acid, alkaline
14. direct, alternating
15. stimulation, irritation

16. vibration
17. stimulating
18. negative
19. rheostat
20. skin, scalp

21. ultra-violet
22. infra-red
23. length, frequency
24. blue
25. red

26. glare, heat
27. 30
28. 12
29. first
30. therapy

TEST 3

DIRECTIONS: In each set of questions, match the items in Column II with the appropriate item in Column I. *PRINT THE LETTER OF THE CORRECT ANSWER IN THE SPACE AT THE RIGHT.*

COLUMN I   COLUMN II

Questions 1-5.

1. Insulator   A. Negatively charged electrical particles   1.____

2. Direct current   B. A substance which conducts an electric current   2.____

3. Electrons   C. A substance which resists the passage of an electric current   3.____

4. Alternating current   D. A current traveling in one direction   4.____

5. Conductor   E. A current traveling first in one direction and then in the opposite direction   5.____

Questions 6-12.

6. Rectifier   A. Pick out the type of required current   6.____

7. Selector switch   B. Regulates current strength   7.____

8. Conducting cords   C. Apply electricity to the body   8.____

9. Rheostat   D. Produce the faradic current   9.____

10. Connecting cords   E. Change an alternating current to a direct current   10.____

11. Induction coil   F. Link wall plate to electric socket   11.____

12. Electrode   G. Carry current from wall plate to electrode   12.____

Questions 13-18.

13. High-frequency current   A. Weak mechanical effect   13.____

14. Galvanic current   B. Strong mechanical effect   14.____

15. Positive pole of galvanic current   C. Increases blood supply   15.____

16. Faradic current   D. Chemical effect   16.____

17. Negative pole of galvanic current   E. Decreases blood supply   17.____

18. Sinusoidal current   F. Thermal effect   18.____

COLUMN I	COLUMN II

Questions 19-30.

19.	A unit of electrical resistance	A. Volt		19._____
20.	A current which has a chemical effect	B. Ohm		20._____
		C. Anode		
21.	A current which is similar to the faradic current	D. Ampere		21._____
		E. Polarity		
		F. Cathode		
22.	An apparatus which changes a direct current to an alternating current	G. Carbon		22._____
		H. Converter		
		I. Sinusoidal current		
23.	The positive terminal of an electric source	J. Ultra-violet rays		23._____
		K. Galvanic current		
24.	The property of having a positive and negative pole	L. Infra-red rays		24._____
		M. Rectifier		
		N. Non-conductor		
25.	Rays emitted from a carbon arc lamp	O. Conductor		25._____
		P. Faradic current		
26.	A unit of electrical pressure			26._____
27.	Rays which have a deep penetrating effect on the skin			27._____
28.	A substance which transmits electricity			28._____
29.	A unit of electrical current			29._____
30.	An asymmetric alternating current			30._____

KEY (CORRECT ANSWERS)

1.	C	16.	A
2.	D	17.	C
3.	A	18.	B
4.	E	19.	B
5.	B	20.	K
6.	E	21.	I
7.	A	22.	H
8.	G	23.	C
9.	B	24.	E
10.	F	25.	J
11.	D	26.	A
12.	C	27.	L
13.	F	28.	O
14.	D	29.	D
15.	E	30.	P